ATLAS OF
EAR KELOIDS

ATLAS OF
EAR KELOIDS
FIRST EDITION

Michael H. Tirgan, MD

Atlas of Ear Keloids

Library of Congress Cataloging-in-Publication Data:
Service Request:

Tirgan, Michael H. 2015

ISBN-13: 978-0-9856553-7-2

Printed in the United States of America.

DEDICATED

to all those who suffer from keloid disorder.

CONTENTS

FORWARD

KELOIDS are an important medical problem which are often under appreciated by the medical community. Dr. Michael Tirgan has spent many years evaluating and treating patients with keloids on different regions of the body. The Atlas of Ear Keloids presents new insights into the natural history of keloids and provides a perspective that many of the standard surgical approaches may actually lead to progression of these tumors on ear. He presents good examples of an alternative treatment with cryotherapy that has convincingly eliminated some of the most troublesome keloids on ear. This book will provide valuable information to patients with keloids on ear and to medical professionals that treat these lesions.

JAMES G. KRUEGER, M.D., PH.D.
Director, Milstein Medical Research Program
Senior Attending Physician
D. Martin Carter Professor in Clinical Investigation
Laboratory of Investigative Dermatology
The Rockefeller University
New York

PREFACE

THIS ATLAS is a compilation of case studies of ear keloids in patients whom I have personally treated. The focus of this book is to review the clinical presentation and natural history of ear keloids.

As you will notice throughout this book, not all ear keloids are the same. Every patient presents with a unique problem. Therefore, the treatment of ear keloids should be customized for each patient. Obviously, the first instinct in a young person who develops ear keloid(s) is to have the keloid(s) surgically removed. As documented throughout this book, rushing into surgery will often result in a worsening of the keloid. A better understanding of some very basic facts will encourage more effective treatment choices.

1 INTRODUCTION

Keloid Is a Genetic Disorder:

KELOID DISORDER is a genetic condition of the skin. Some individuals are born with a propensity to develop keloids. In addition to the genetic predisposition to develop keloids, there must be an injury to the skin that would trigger abnormal wound healing processes. The underlying genetics of keloid disorder are not well understood. There appears to be a spectrum to this genetic predisposition, supported by the fact that some individuals suffer from a very mild form of this condition, and others from a moderate to severe form of this disorder.

On one end of the spectrum, we observe patients who develop very few and small keloids. There are also individuals who develop a keloid only after sustaining a major injury to their skin, such as surgery for the treatment of a medical condition, or a surgical facelift as they age. There are also those who, despite carrying the genes, never develop a keloid and remain as *asymptomatic carriers*. These are the parents of keloid patients who have never developed a keloid themselves, or siblings who don't develop keloids at all.

On the other end of the keloid genetic spectrum, there are patients with a very severe form of this disorder who will develop several large keloids on different parts of their skin. Their keloids grow over time and remain refractory to our current treatments.

Keloid Involves Patches of Skin

Clinical observation of keloid patients supports the hypothesis that keloid disorder only involves certain parts of the skin. There are numerous patients who have had prior injuries to various parts of their skin, yet keloid formation has been limited to certain areas. This fact, compounded by (1) the genetic spectrum of the severity of the disorder and (2) the severity of the injury to the skin, leads to a highly variable presentation of the illness among the sufferers of this disorder.

If there was a scientific method to map the skin of keloid patients in order to determine the parts of the skin that are prone to developing keloids, that map would show only certain patches of the skin being prone, and other areas being spared from the disorder.

Furthermore, every keloid patient does have his or her own unique map that is different from other patients. A clear example of the patchy involvement of the skin in keloid disorder is seen among patients with ear keloids who, after piercing both ears, develop a keloid on one side only; or among those who undergo otoplasty surgery on both ears, yet develop a keloid on only one side. To that end, the intensity of genetic predisposition to keloid formation may also vary in each patch of the skin.

Some patients develop keloids on both ears, yet the keloids are not symmetrical and differ in their size and growth rate.

The Nature of Keloid Disorder

Although keloid disorder has been recognized for many centuries, very little research has been done into its biology, genetics and variable behavioral patterns. The culprit in the formation of keloidal lesions is the wounding of the skin in genetically prone individuals.

Disruption in the normal anatomy of the skin and subsequent genetically driven dysregulated wound healing processes lead to the formation of keloid lesions. Wound healing is a very complex and dynamic process that normally results in restoration of the anatomy and function of the skin. A normal and balanced wound healing response results in minimal scar formation. Keloid formation, on the other hand, is due to an uninhibited, excessive and prolonged wound healing response to a dermal injury; as if the brakes on the wound healing process were malfunctioning.

The result is an excessive healing response and deposition of collagen that outgrows the original site of the skin injury.

Ear Keloids:

The ears are common locations for the development of keloids. The injury that triggers ear keloid formation is almost always due to piercing.

The second most common type of injury to the ear is surgery, either to remove a previously formed keloid, or surgery for other reasons, such as otoplasty to reshape the ears, or facelift surgery.

The worsening of earlobe keloids after surgical excision is most definitely due to triggering the underlying dysregulated wound healing mechanisms. This is in response to a new, yet greater, dermal injury—i.e. surgery—which is more extensive in nature than the original piercing injury.

The age of onset for the development of keloid peaks during puberty and the early teens. It is therefore postulated that, although the genetic susceptibility is transmitted from parents to their children, the actual disorder is not triggered until children reach puberty.

The most captivating case I have encountered was a young African American female who had keloids in both her ears. Her earlobes were pierced when she was very little. It was only when she was between fifteen and sixteen years of age when she first noticed keloids forming on her earlobes at the sites of her old piercings.

Psycho-Social Impacts of Ear Keloids:

Despite their benign nature, ear keloids may constitute a severe aesthetic and, in some cases, functional problem with important repercussions.

We can safely assume this of ear keloids, in particular, since they are visible and can impact the overall performance of patients in society. The psycho-social impact of the primary keloids is often less severe, as patients have high hopes for a cure.

This hope vanishes with the recurrence of keloids after surgery and the formation of a new, and larger keloid.

Anxiety and depression are natural human reactions to chronic disorders such as keloid. Disfigurement of the ear after surgery, and unsightly recurrent keloids, diminish the quality of life of almost every patient, and become psychologically devastating for some.

2 PRIMARY EAR KELOIDS

A *PRIMARY EAR keloid* is a keloid that has not been previously treated with surgery. Keloid lesions can form in any part of the ear, however. The location of the keloid mostly depends upon the site of the prior piercing.

All primary ear keloids start as a small skin lesion and grow over time. The longer a keloid is present, the larger it will become. The images presented below show primary keloids in different stages of development.

The rate of growth of ear keloids that form in the same anatomical location varies among individuals. This is perhaps due to variability in the genetics of this disorder.

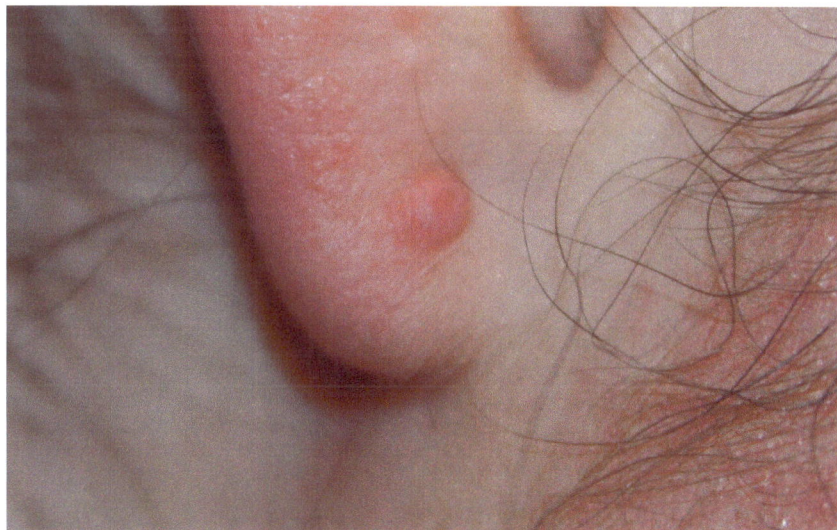

Fig. 1: A small keloid on the frontal side of the right earlobe. This is the earliest evidence of the development of a keloid after ear piercing.

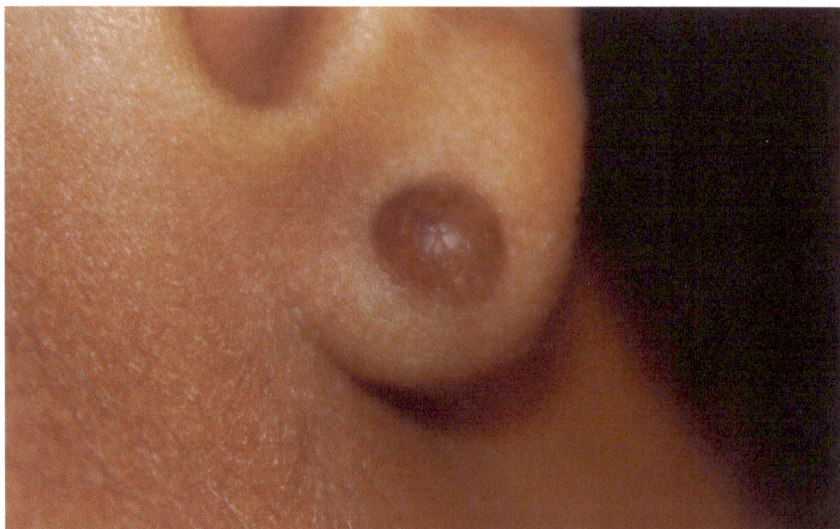

Fig. 2: A small keloid on the frontal side of the left earlobe.

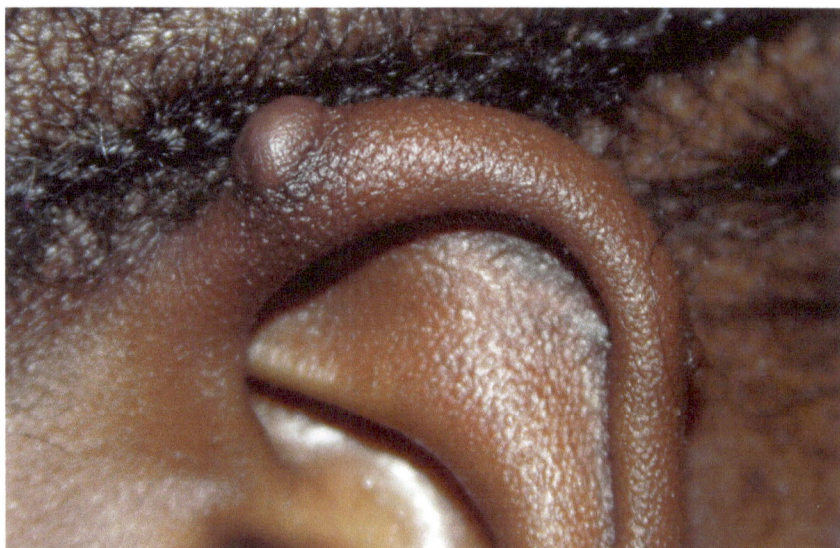

Fig. 3: Two small keloids have formed on the helix of the left ear at both sides of a cross bar piercing.

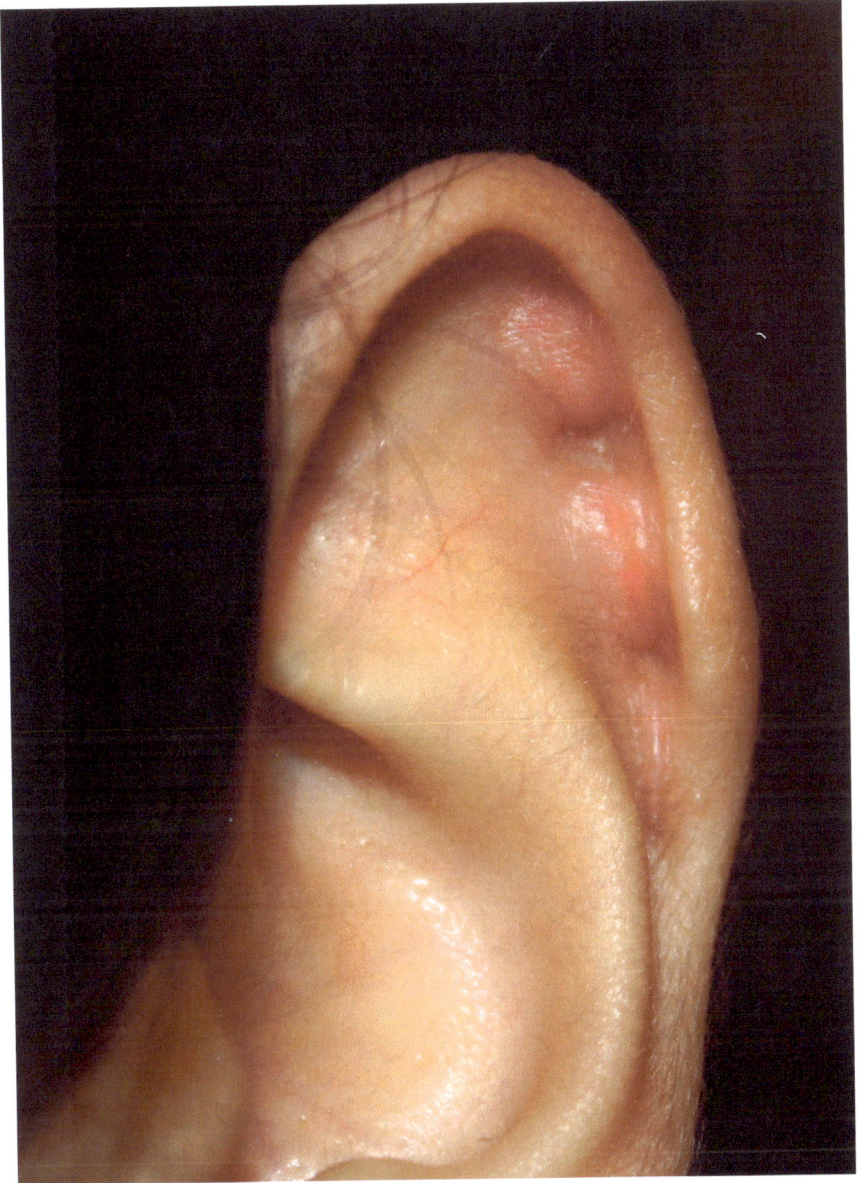

Fig. 4: Three distinct small areas of keloid formation around pierced sites.

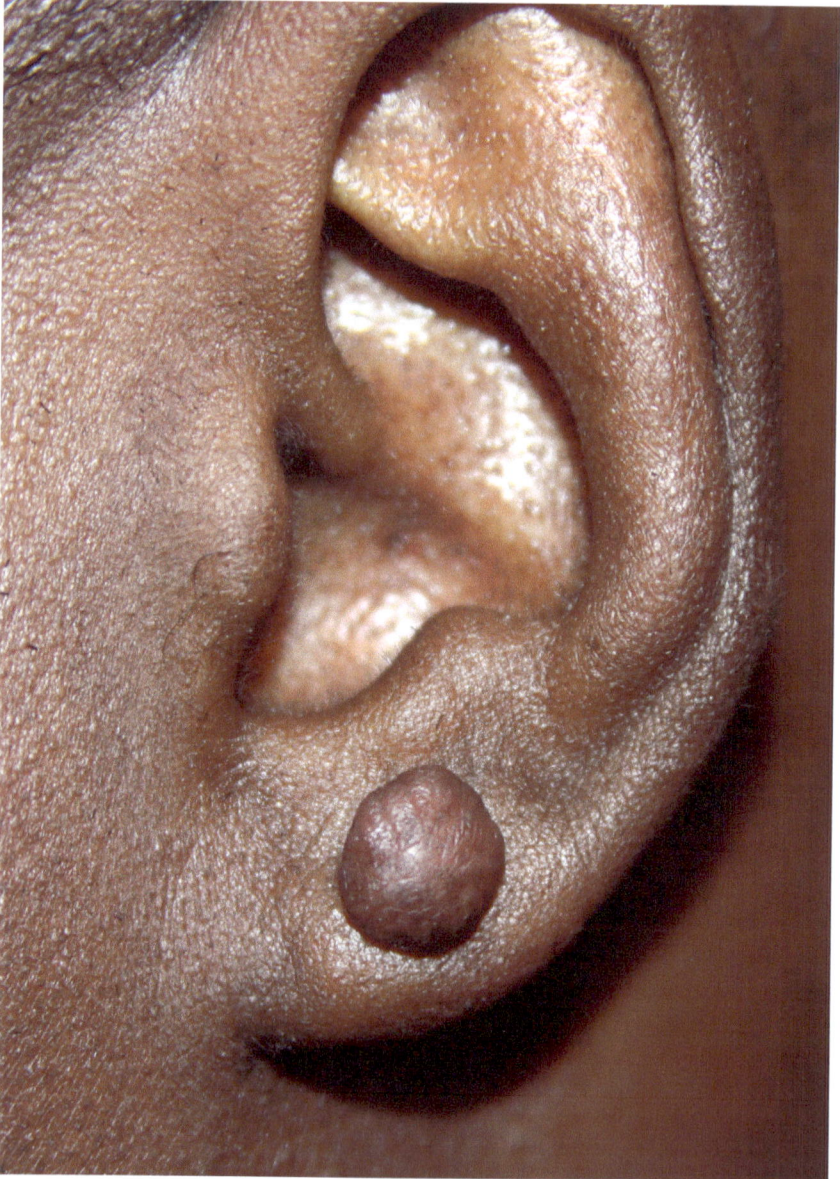

Fig. 5: An early stage, small size primary earlobe keloid at the site of an earlobe piercing.

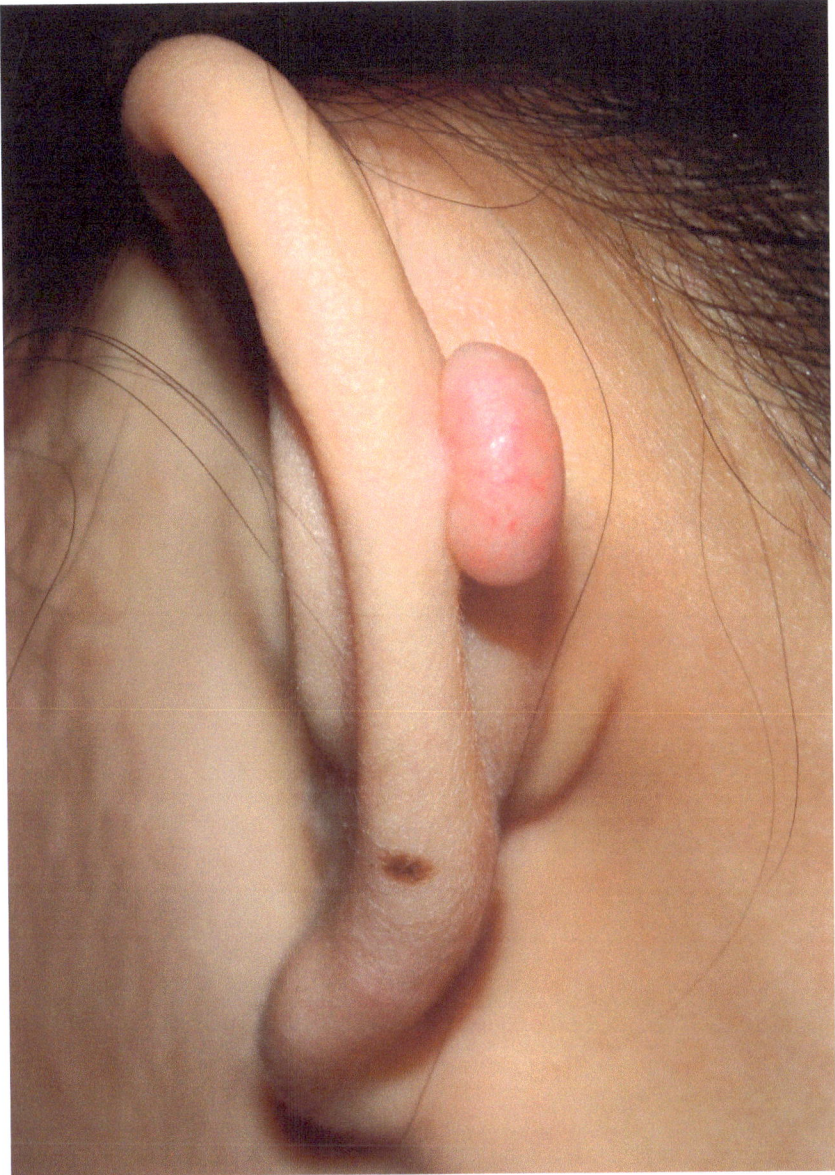

Fig. 6: An early stage primary keloid of the ear that has formed on only one side of the ear, despite the fact that the piercing injury has damaged both surfaces of the ear.

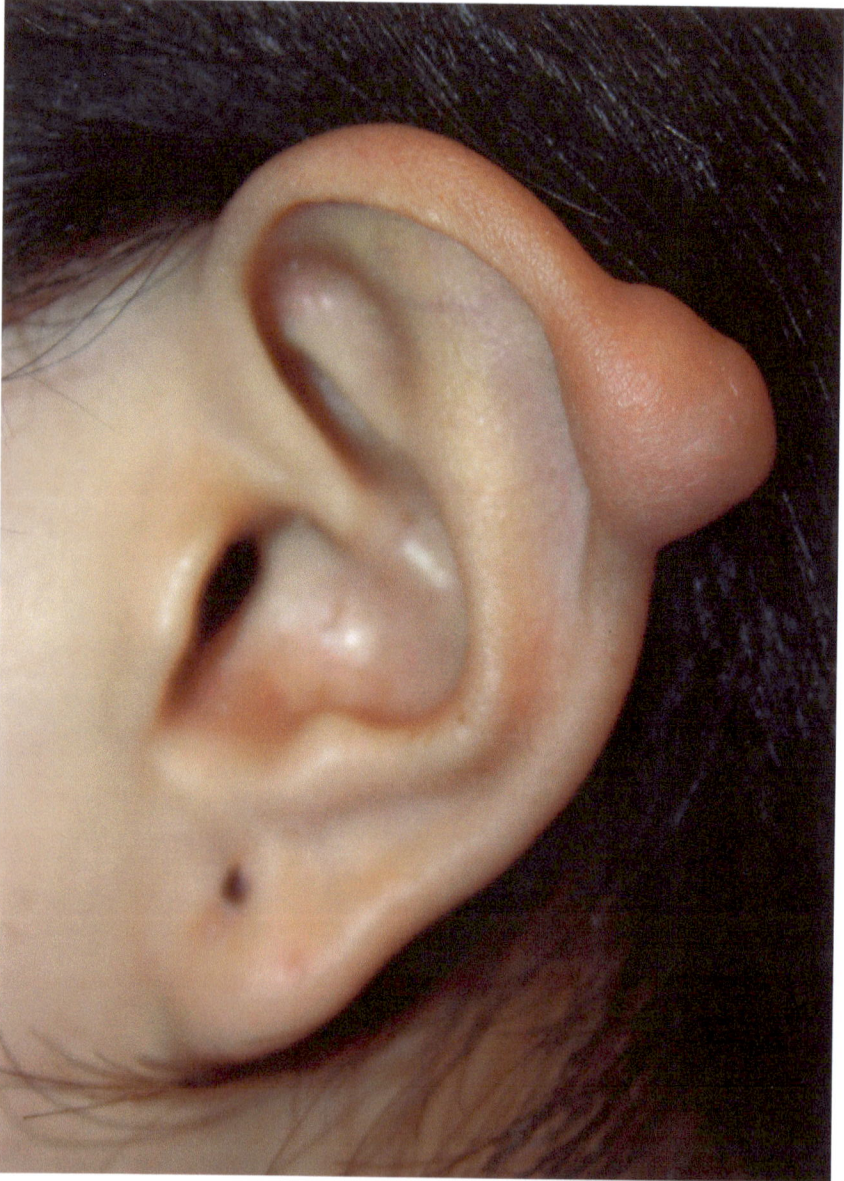

Fig. 7: An early stage single primary ear keloid of the left ear that has involved both surfaces of the helix.

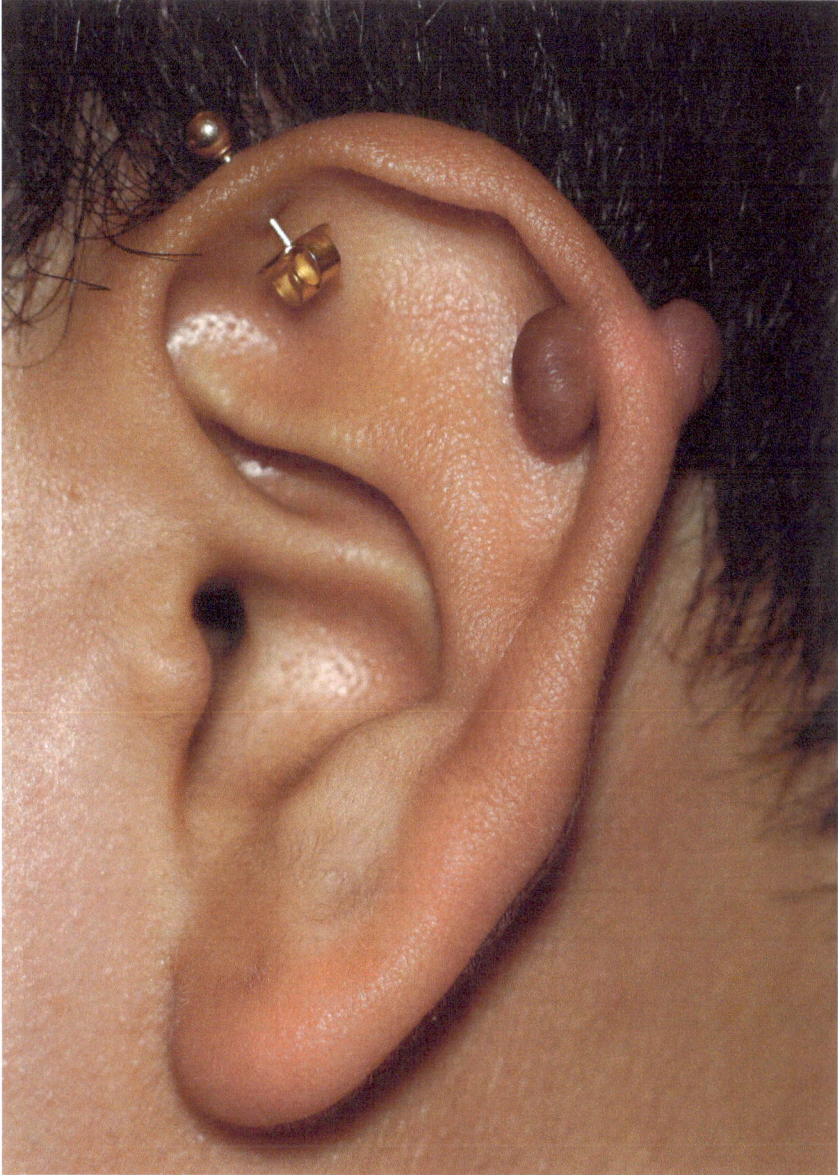

Fig. 8: Two small keloids have formed on both sides of one pierced spot.

This patient had a cross bar ear piercing but, rather interestingly, she developed keloids on only one piercing site. As discussed earlier, not all areas of the skin are prone to developing keloids.

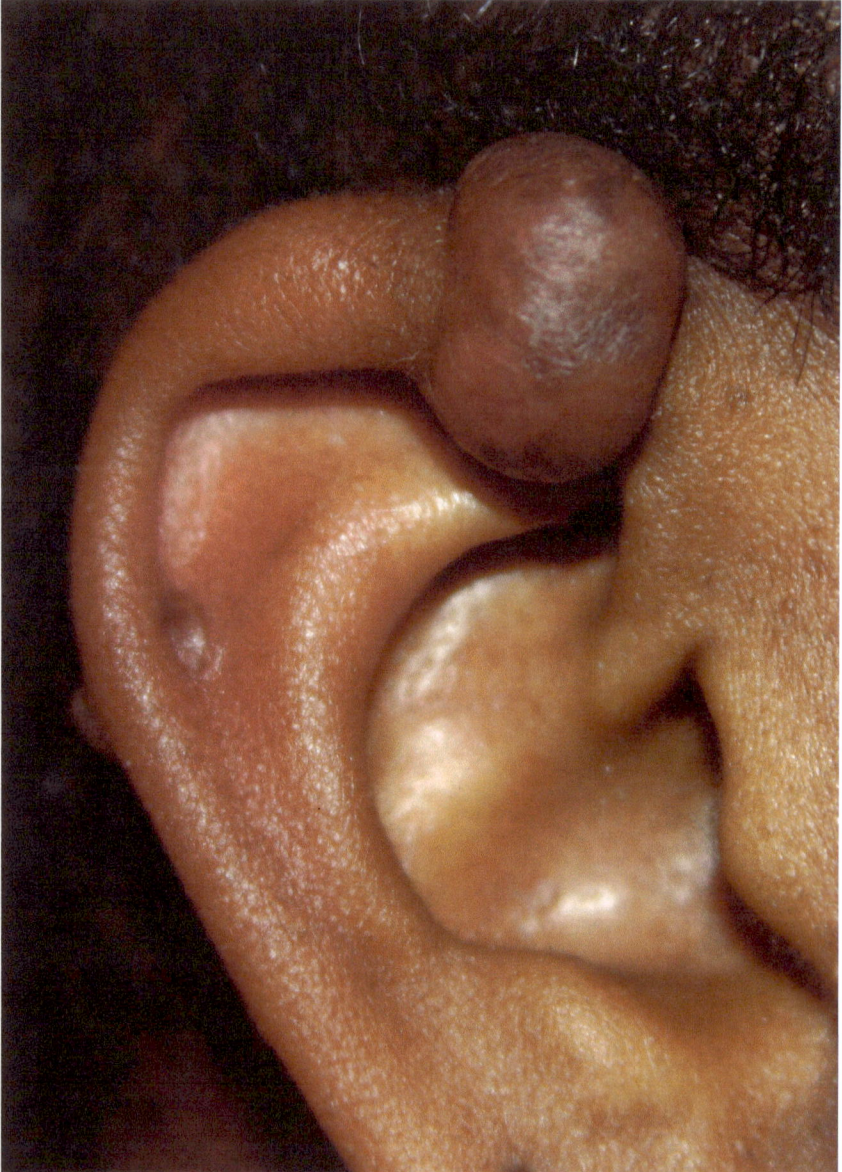

Fig. 9: Primary ear keloids that vary in size and shape formed after a crossbar piercing of the helix of the ear.

Keloids that form on different surfaces of a pierced site may or may not maintain the same rate of growth, shape or size.

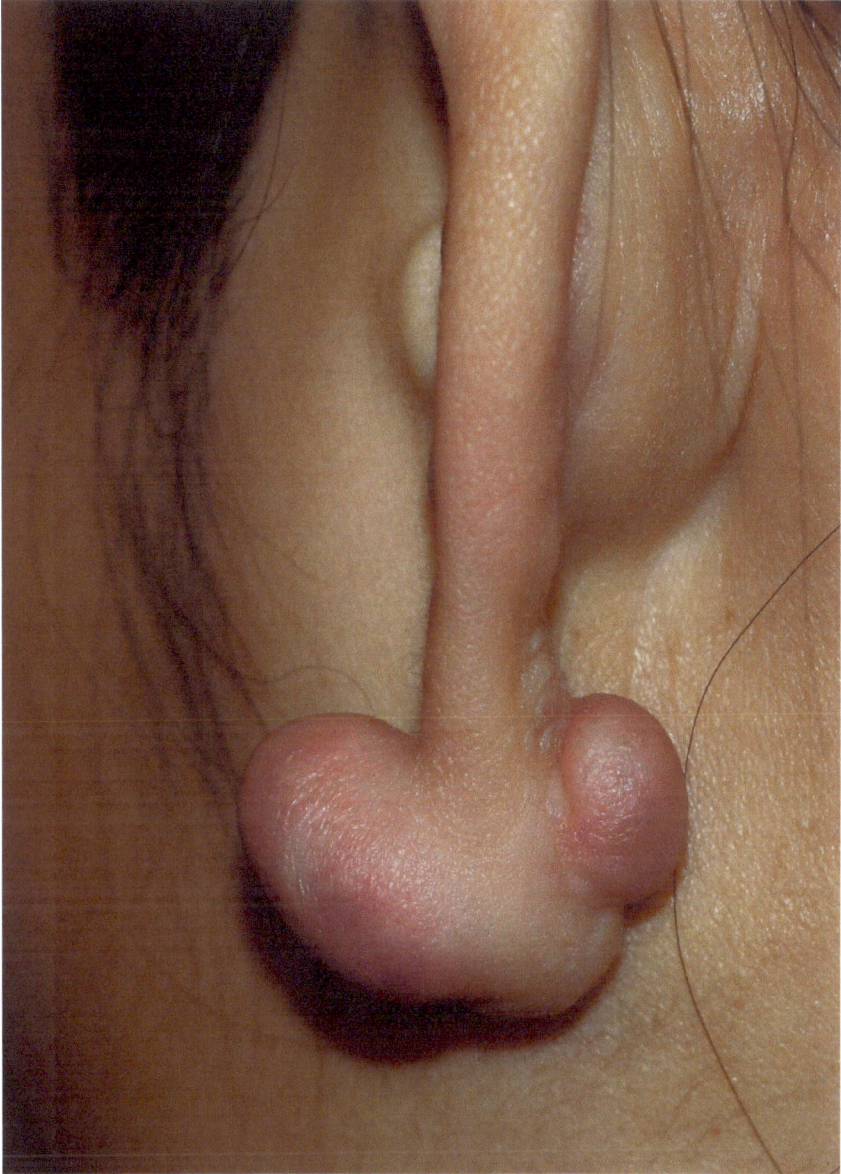

Fig. 10: Two keloids, different in size and shape, formed on both sides of the earlobe.

As time passes, primary ear keloids grow in size at rates that vary among different individuals. In some cases, the keloids tend to grow very slowly and remain small in size. In others, keloids can grow rather quickly and become larger in a shorter time frame.

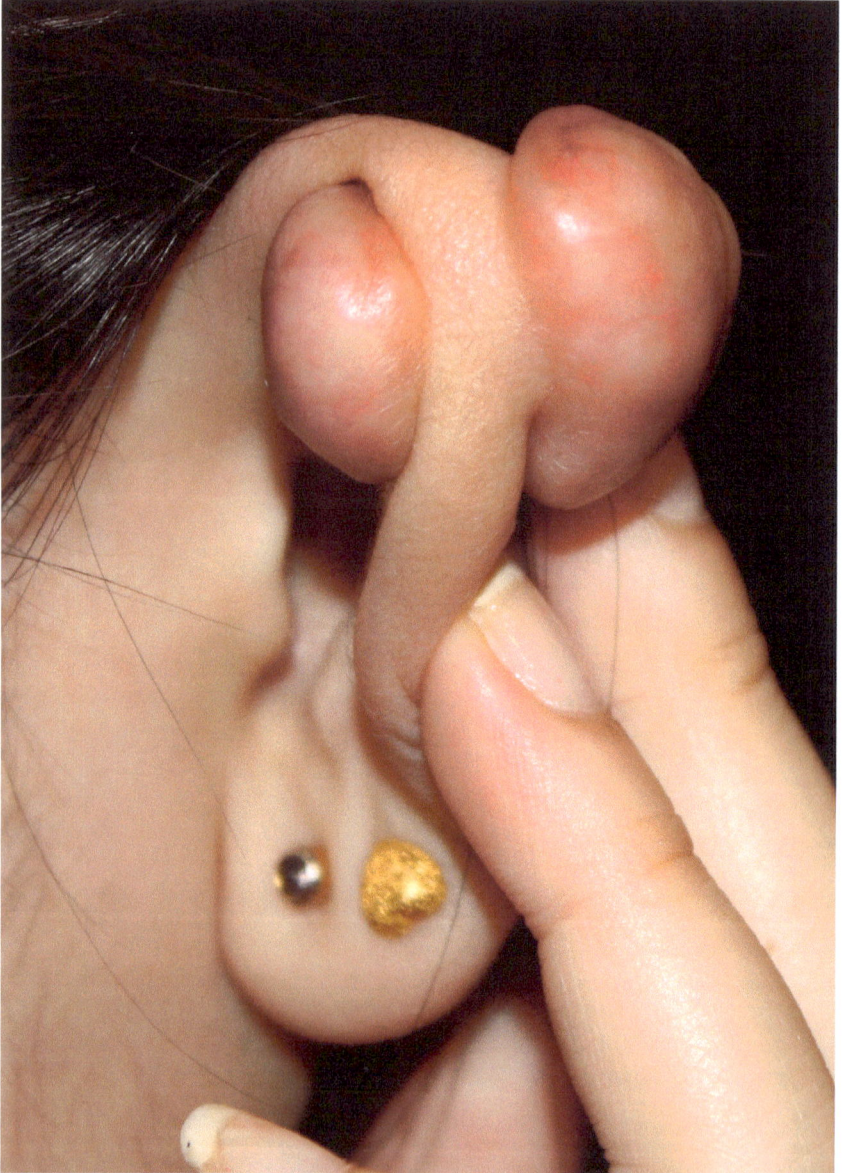

Fig. 11: Primary ear keloids that have formed on both surfaces of the helix with variable rates of growth and variable sizes and shapes.

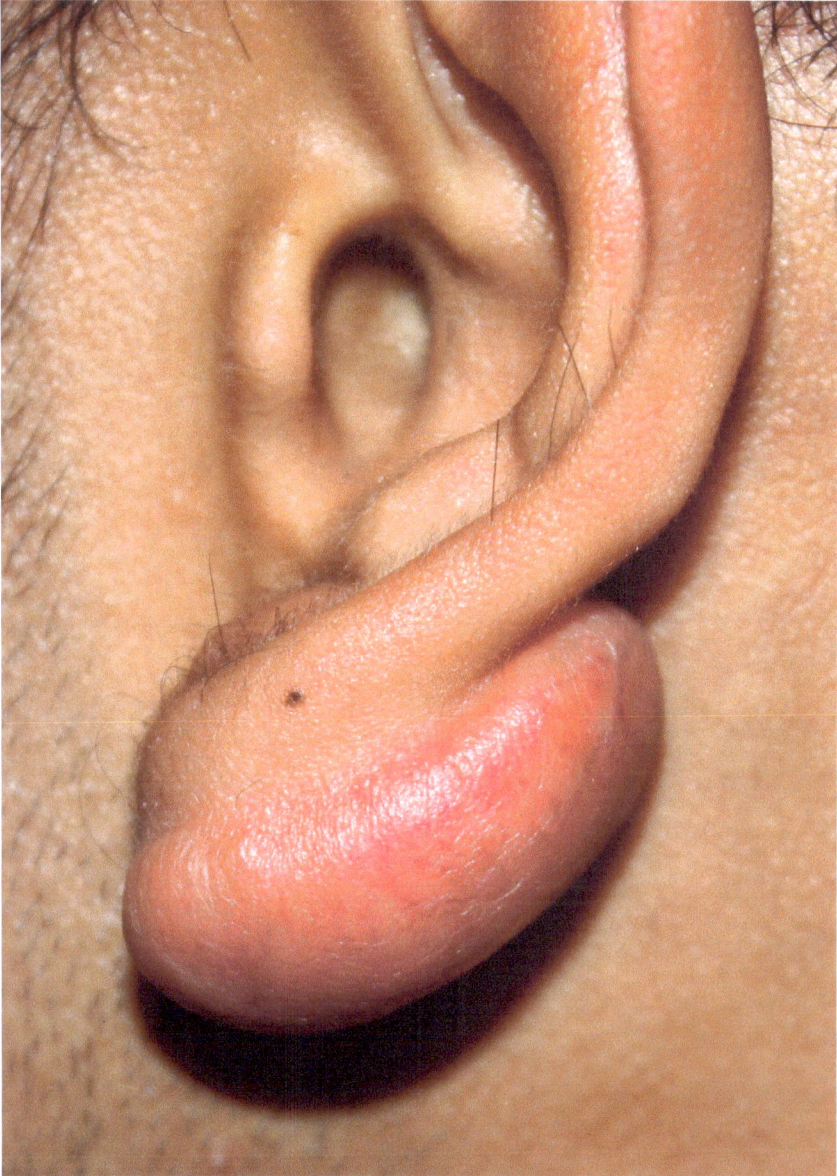

Fig. 12: A primary keloid of the earlobe that has grown only on one side of the earlobe.

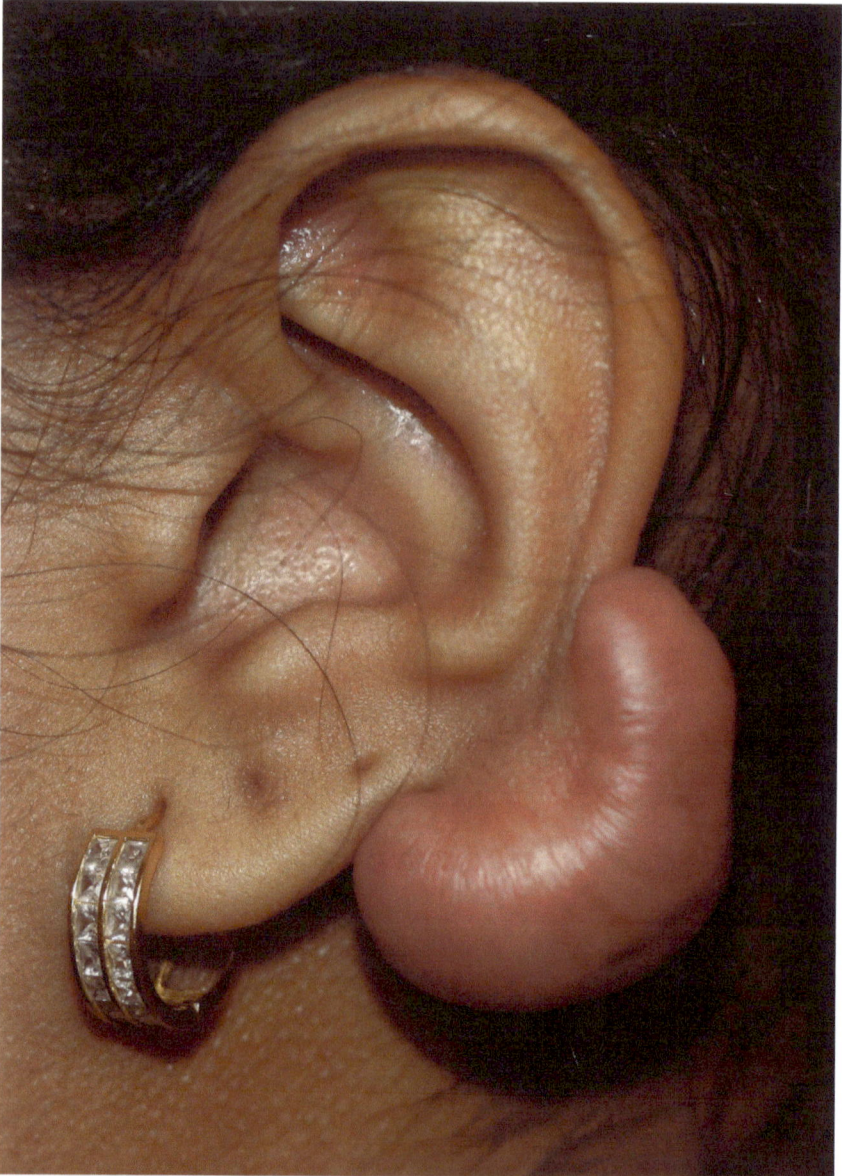

Fig. 13: A primary ear keloid. Notice that this patient has several piercing sites, yet has developed a keloid only on one site.

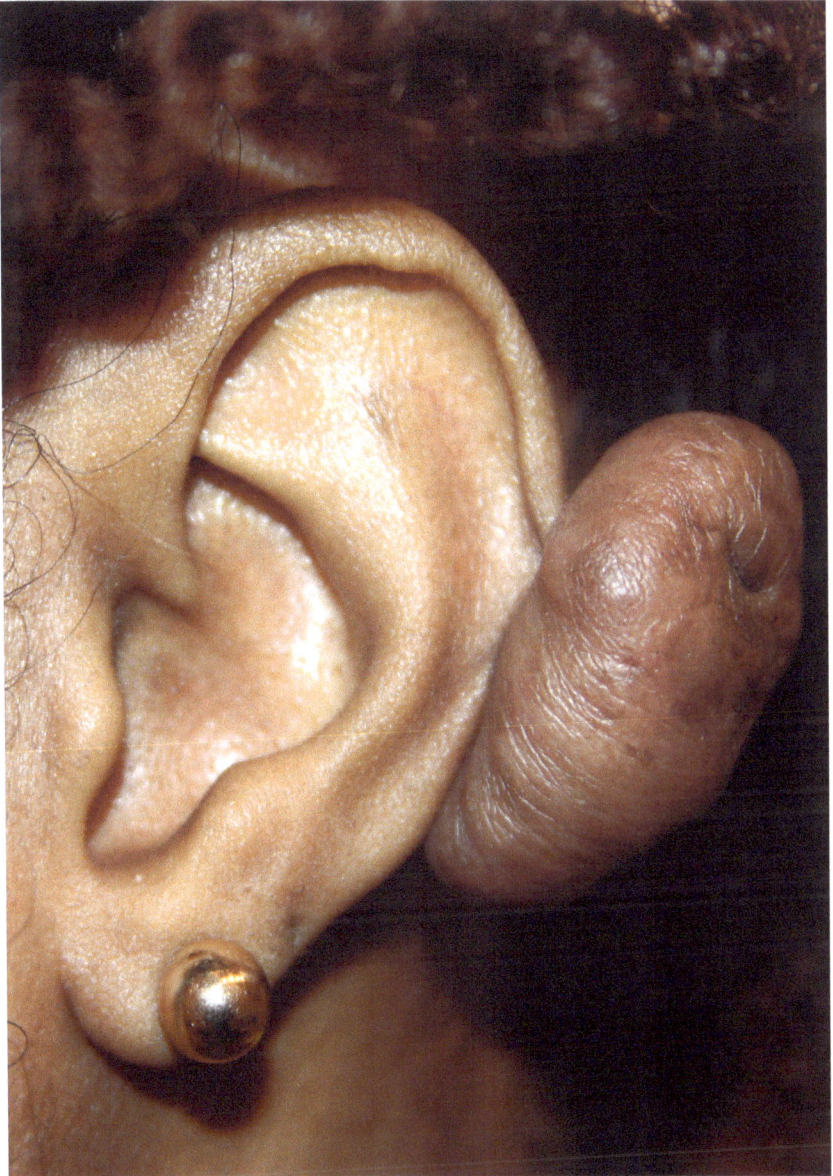

Fig. 14: A primary ear keloid. Notice that this patient also has several piercing sites, yet has developed a keloid only on one site.

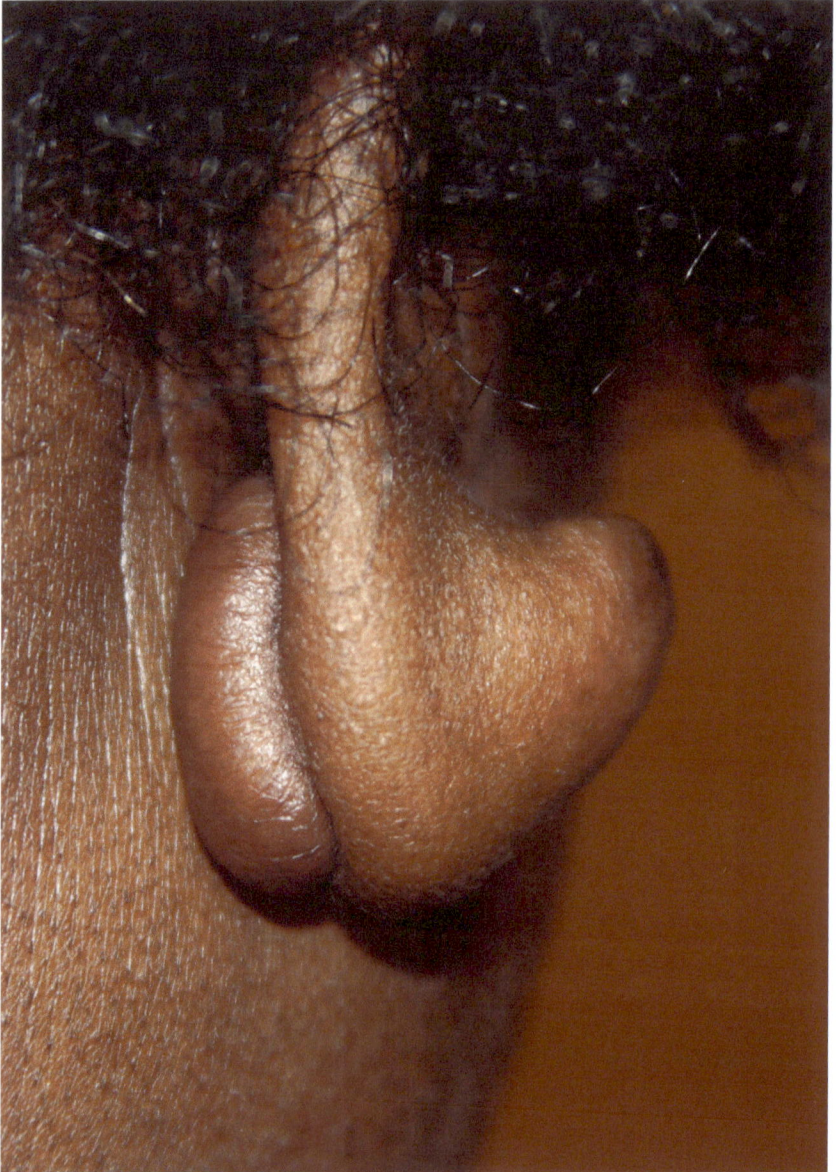

Fig. 15: Primary keloids of the earlobe involving the whole thickness of the right earlobe. Some keloids grow through the full thickness of the earlobe.

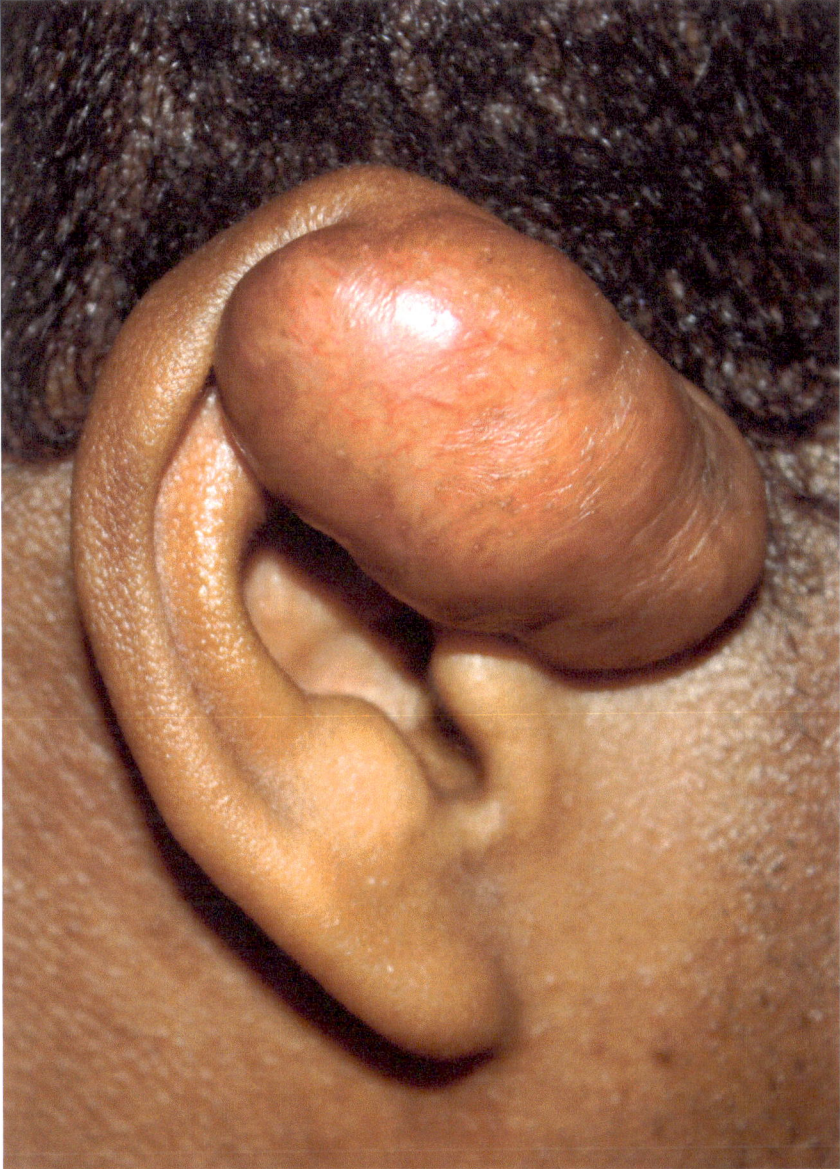

Fig. 16: A large primary keloid of the helix.

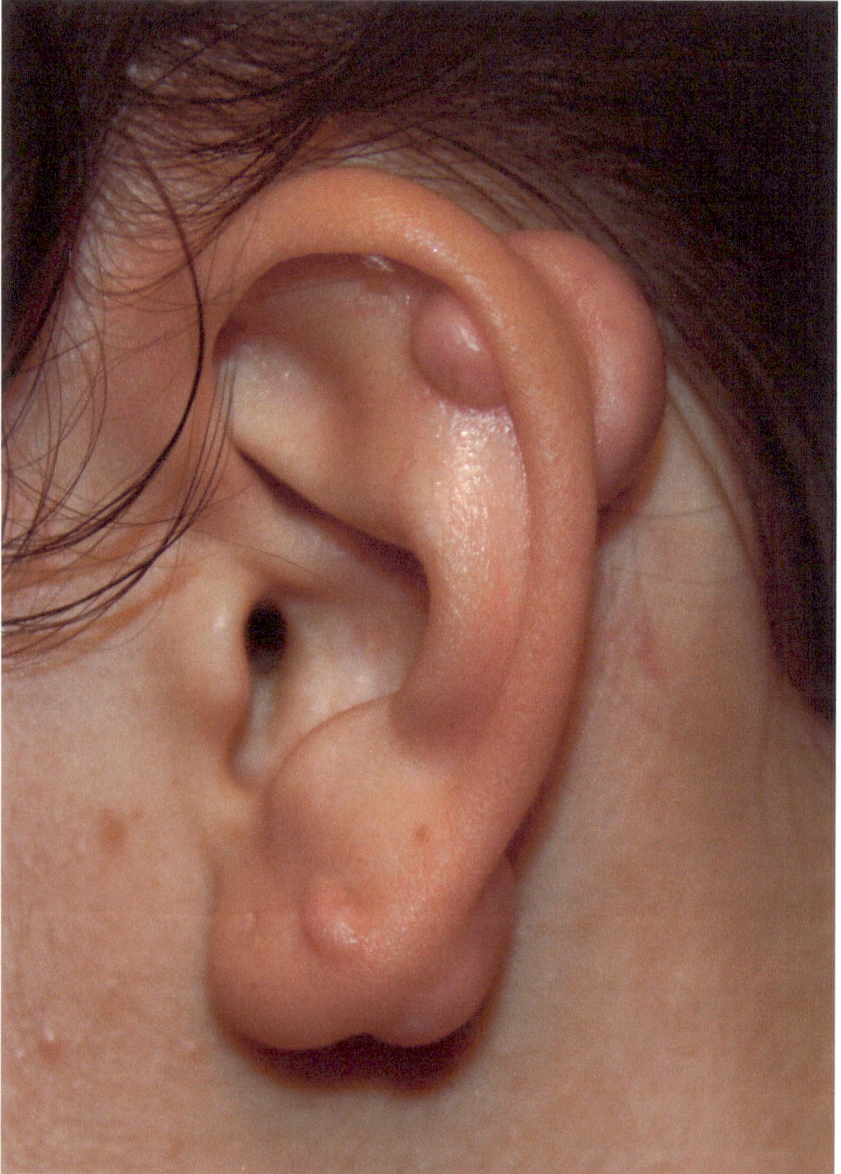

Fig. 17: Primary keloids that have formed on both piercing sites. Please notice that all four keloids are unique in their shapes.

3 Aftermath of Surgery

THE GOAL OF treatment for any keloid, and ear keloids in particular, should not only pivot on removal of the keloid tissue but, most importantly, on two very crucial principles:

1. Prevention of damage to the ear
2. Prevention of the recurrence of keloid

Performing surgery to remove primary ear keloids is inherently contrary to these two very basic principles. Surgery by its nature induces a totally new injury to the skin of the ear. Quite often, surgical removal of a primary keloid also results in the loss of surrounding normal ear tissue. Loss of normal ear tissue, even in the absence of future keloid recurrence, will result in an unacceptable esthetic outcome.

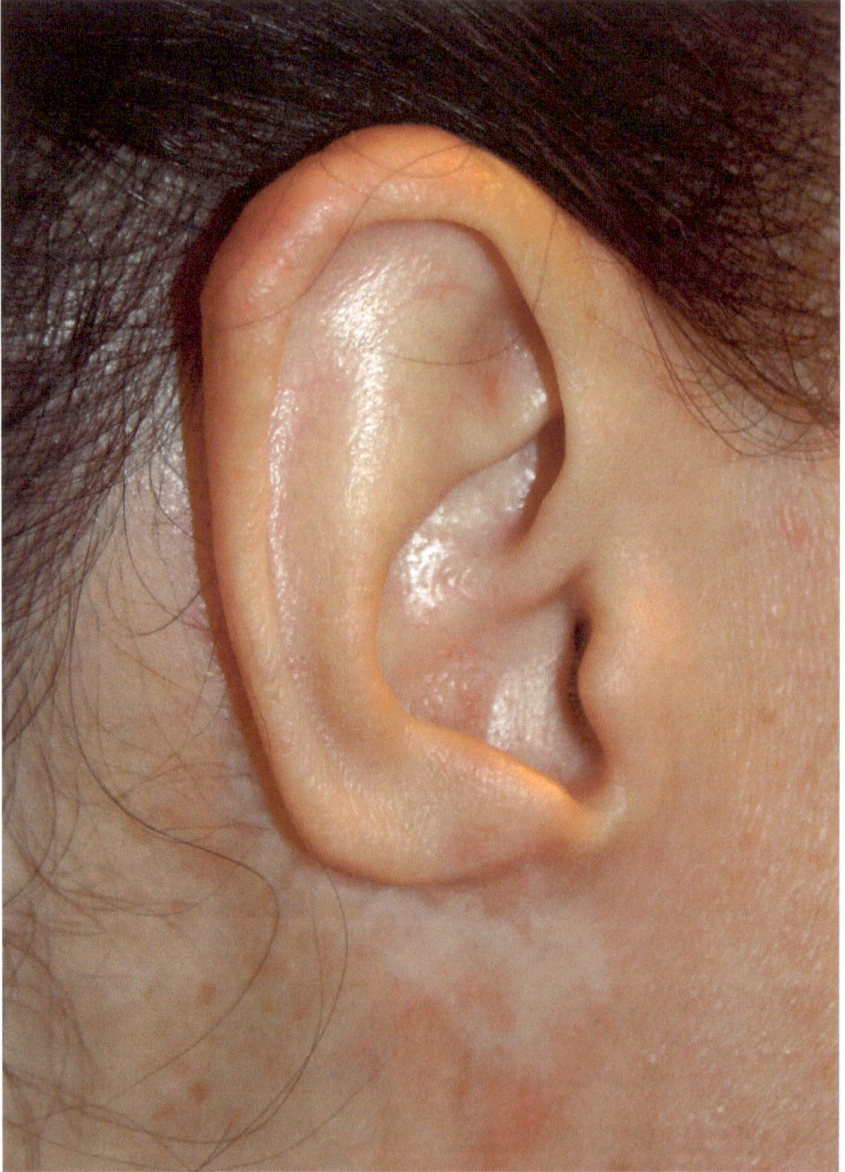

Fig. 18: Total loss of earlobe tissue and disfigurement of the ear after surgery to remove earlobe keloid. This expected negative outcome is often downplayed prior to surgery.

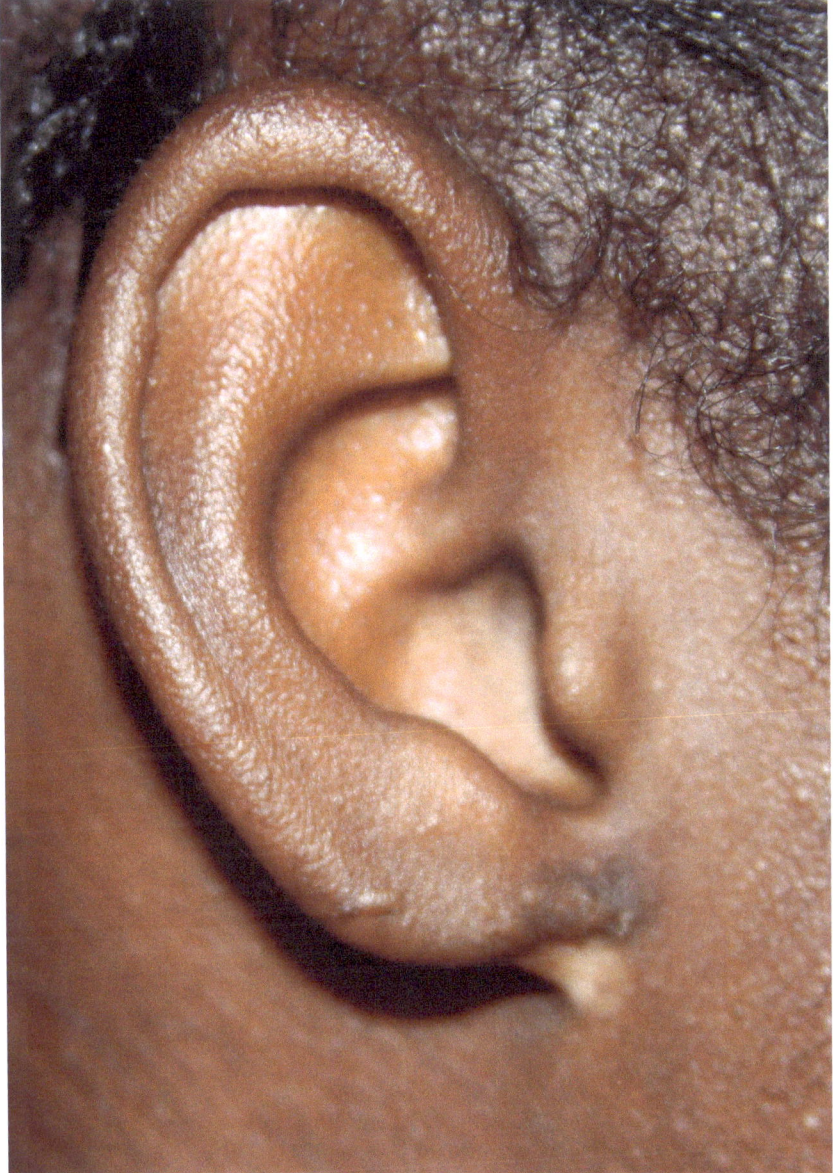

Fig. 19: Total loss of earlobe tissue after surgery in a seventeen year-old female. Patients like this young woman will suffer from this disfigurement even in the absence of recurrence of keloid.

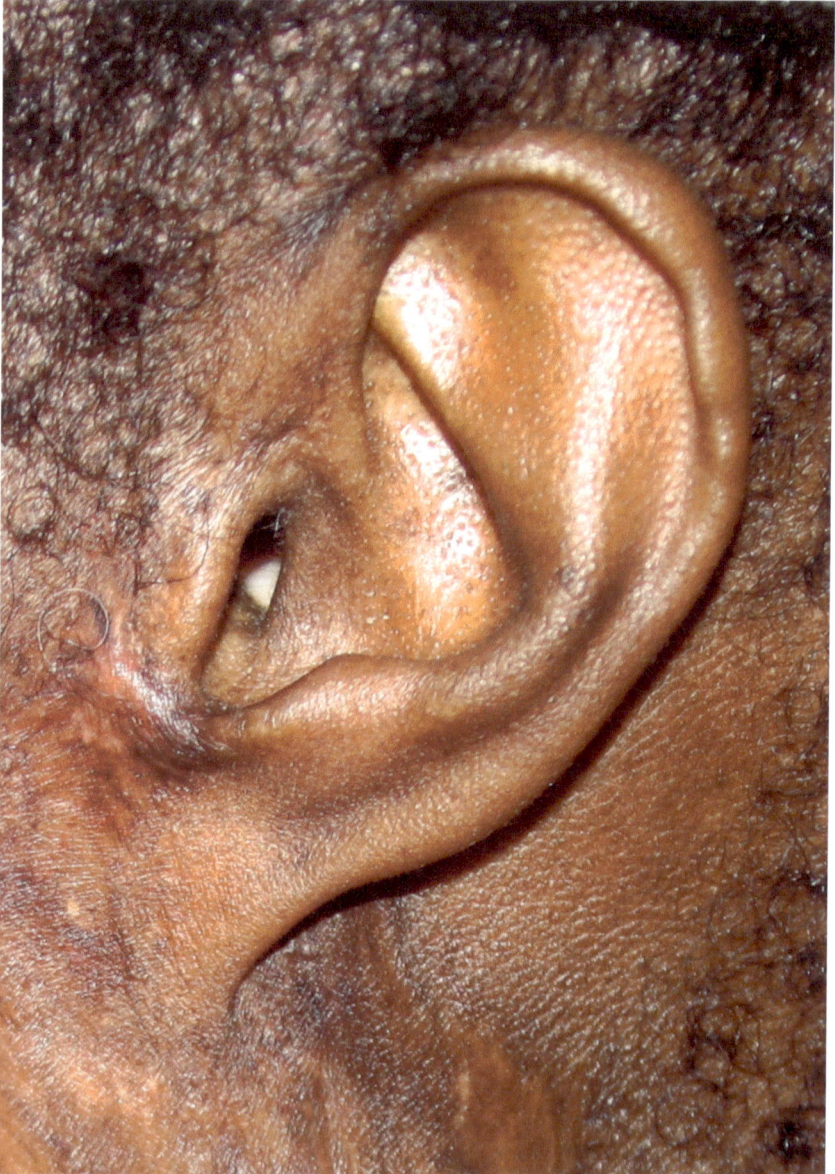

Fig. 20: Loss of earlobe tissue and disfigurement of ear after surgery in a young woman.

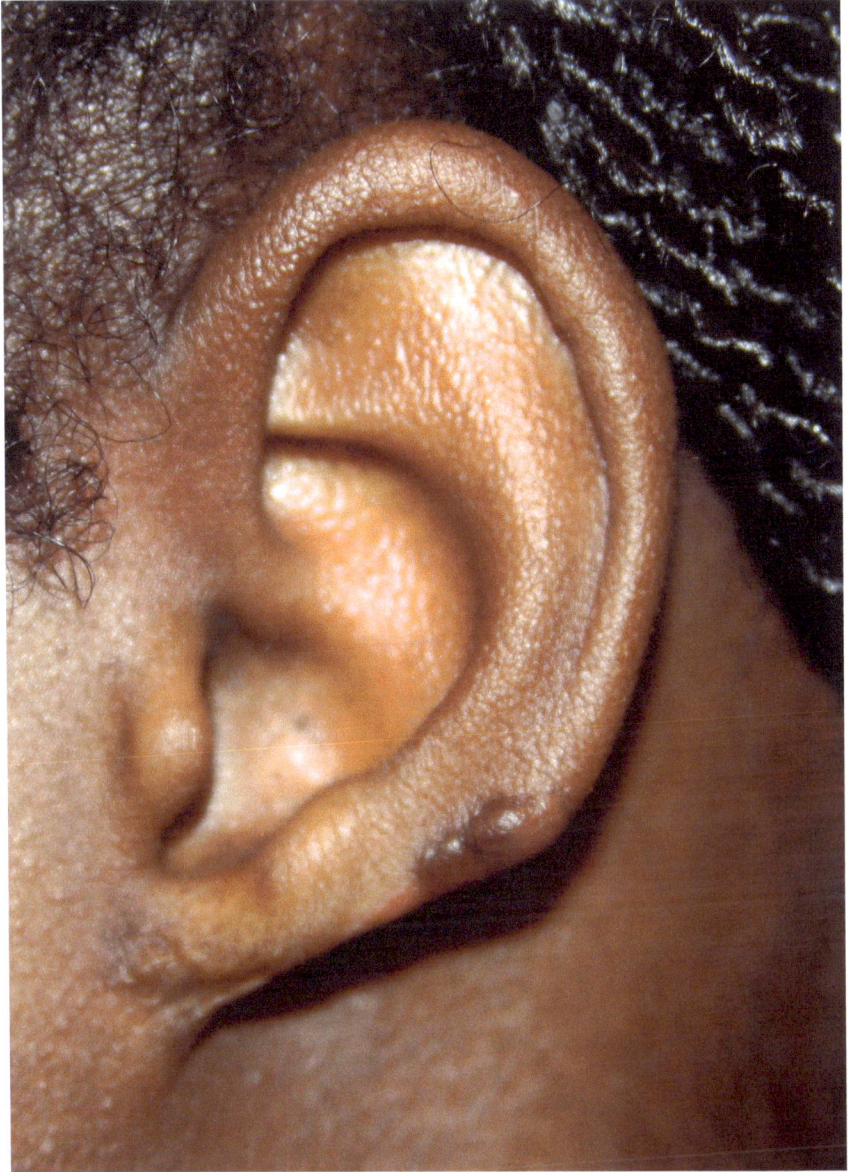

Fig. 21: Total loss of earlobe tissue after surgery.

What is most disturbing in this case is that the disfiguring surgery did not resolve the keloid process. There is clear evidence of the recurrence of the keloid just above the site of surgery. The most unfortunate scenario is recurrence of the keloid, despite the loss of normal ear tissue.

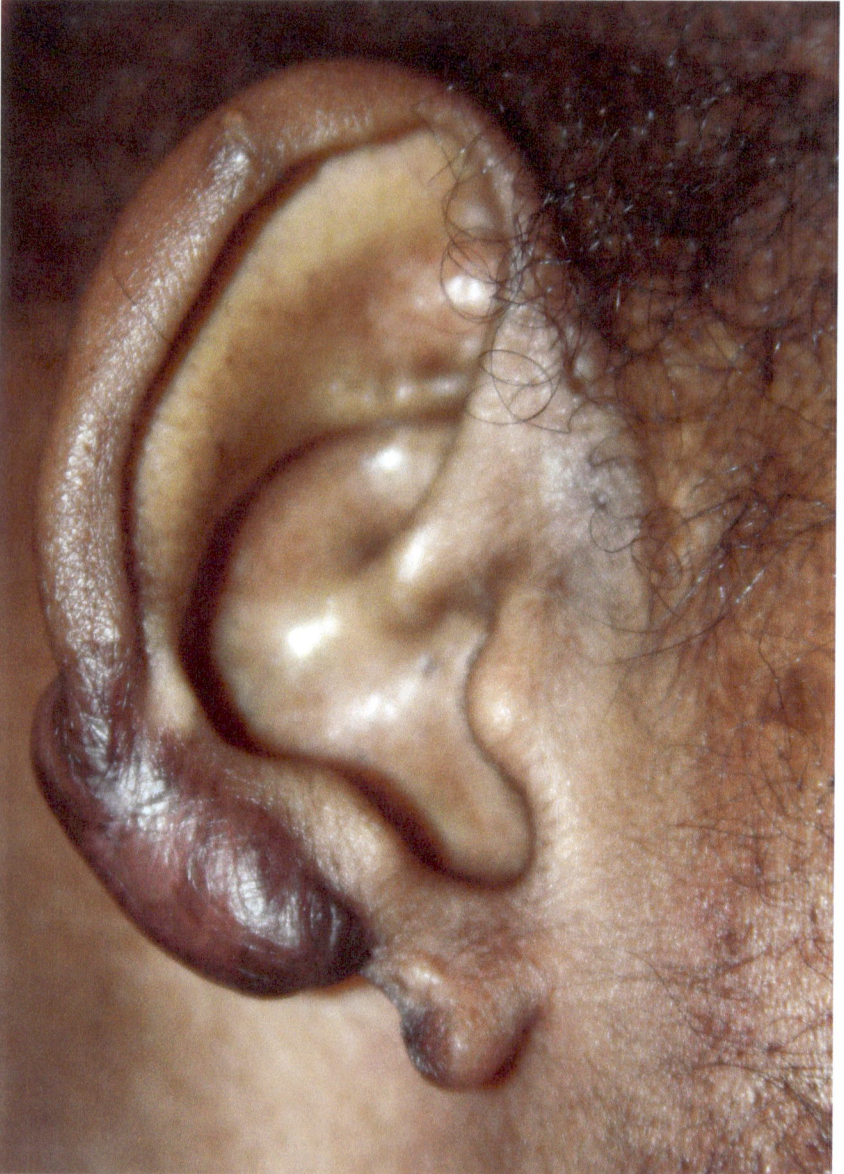

Fig. 22: Recurrence of the keloid, in addition to the near-total loss of earlobe tissue after surgery.

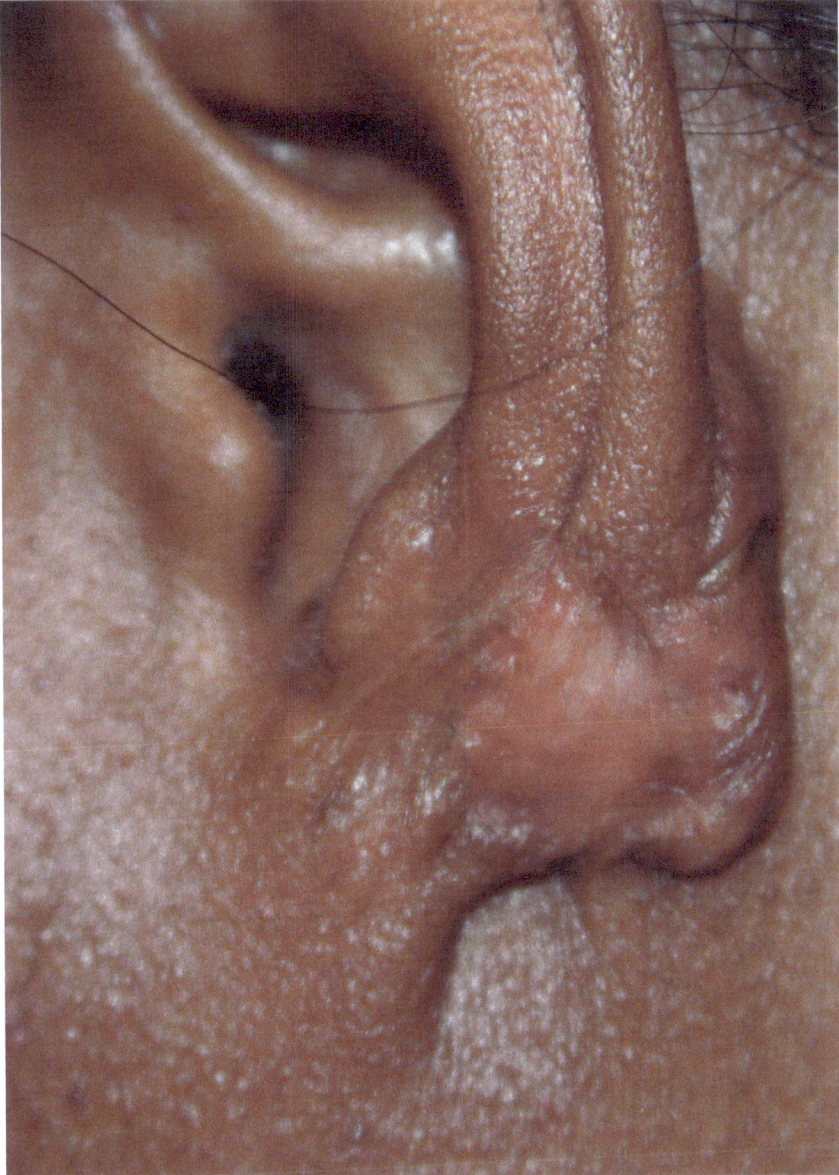

Fig. 23: Recurrence of the keloid at the site of a prior surgery in addition to total loss of earlobe tissue after surgery.

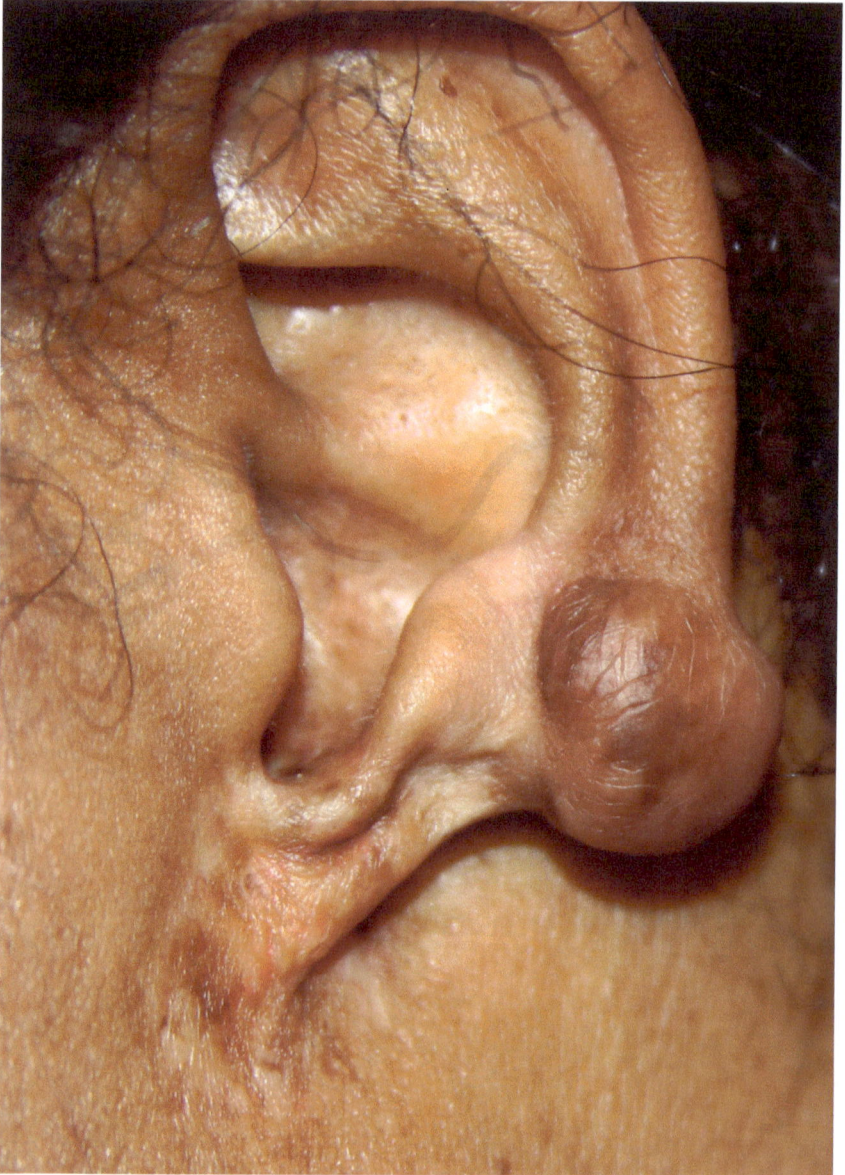

Fig. 24: Recurrence of the keloid at the site of prior surgery in addition to total loss of earlobe tissue after surgery.

4 SECONDARY EAR KELOIDS

A *SECONDARY KELOID* is a new keloid that forms at the site of a surgery for the removal of a primary keloid. Since the extent of injury to the ear from surgery is significantly more than the injury from piercing, all patients who undergo surgery are at risk of developing new, larger keloids at the site of surgery.

By far, the most important principle to follow in treating all primary ear keloids is to refrain from surgery at all costs. Cognizant of the fact that there are some patients whose keloids do not recur after surgery, we must be well aware of the nightmare that many other patients have to deal with due to the recurrence of their ear keloid after surgery.

The psychological stress and anxiety that a young person is put through by having to live with a worsened keloid is real and life changing.

The size and appearance of secondary keloids depends on the extent and location of the surgical wound. Secondary keloids tend to grow faster than their primary counterparts. If left untreated, secondary keloids can grow to a very large size and can deform the whole ear. The following images depict a wide range of secondary keloids.

Indiscriminate and repeated surgical attempts to remove ear keloids is associated with several issues.

1. **The recurrence rate** after surgery to remove a keloid is nearly 100 percent. The reason for such a high recurrence rate is obviously the genetic abnormality of the skin, which will not

change with surgery and which will be present throughout the life of the person. Several practices are used to reduce the recurrence rate; such as injecting the site of surgery with steroids, or using pressure earrings or radiation, all with varied and often unsatisfactory outcomes. Recurrent keloids, if left untreated, become larger and more complex than the corresponding primary keloids. Very large keloids of the ear form exclusively after failed surgical attempts to remove a primary, or a secondary keloid. As depicted earlier in this book, primary ear keloids hardly ever reach the size and shape of secondary keloids.

2. **The impairment** of the actual ear shape due to surgery, or due to the development of very large keloids, is another iatrogenic problem that is imposed on some patients. Quite often, in an effort to remove the whole keloid, the surgeon removes part of the ear, or performs a wedge resection of the keloid and the tissue adjacent to the keloid. This approach, if it does not lead to the recurrence of the keloid, which it often does, will result in the loss of normal ear tissue, the disturbance of normal ear anatomy and a poor esthetic outcome.

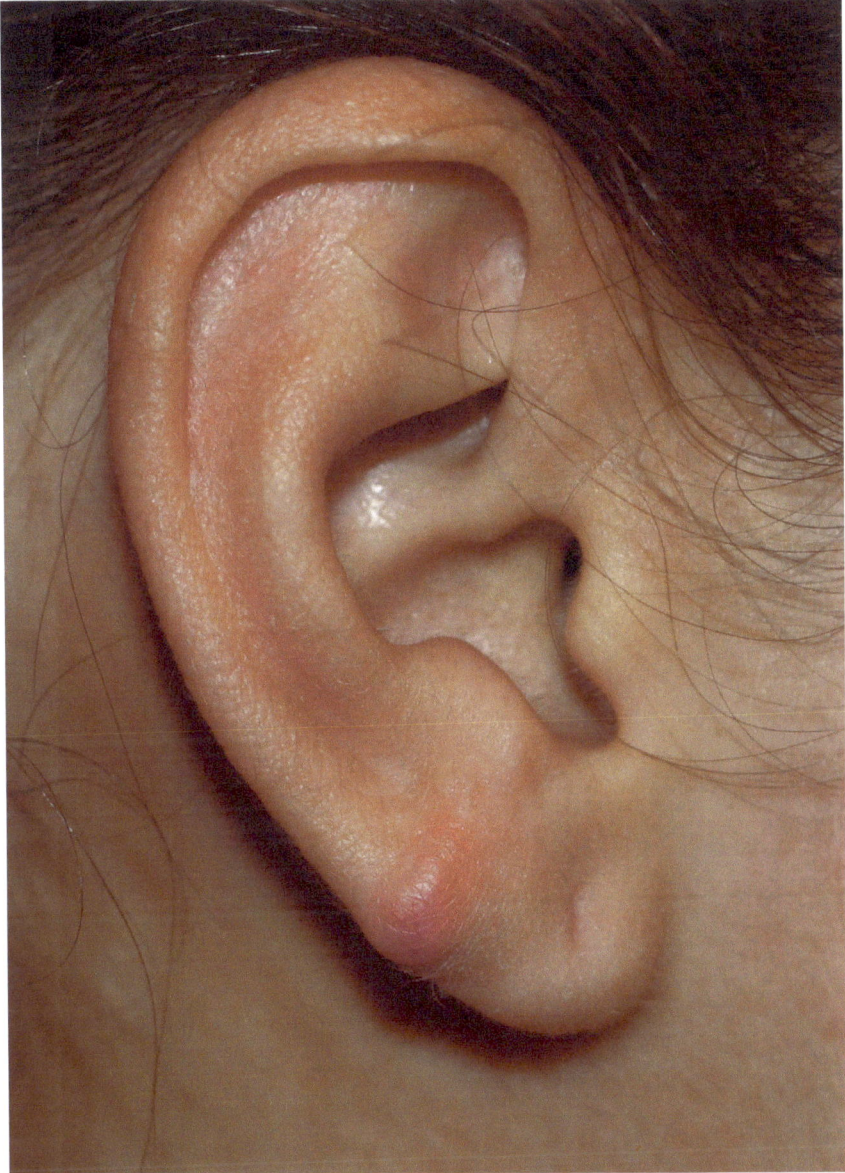

Fig. 25: A small secondary earlobe keloid in a young female. This earlobe keloid was previously removed surgically by a wedge resection of the portion of the ear that contained the keloid. This patient is presented in an early stage of her recurrent secondary keloid.

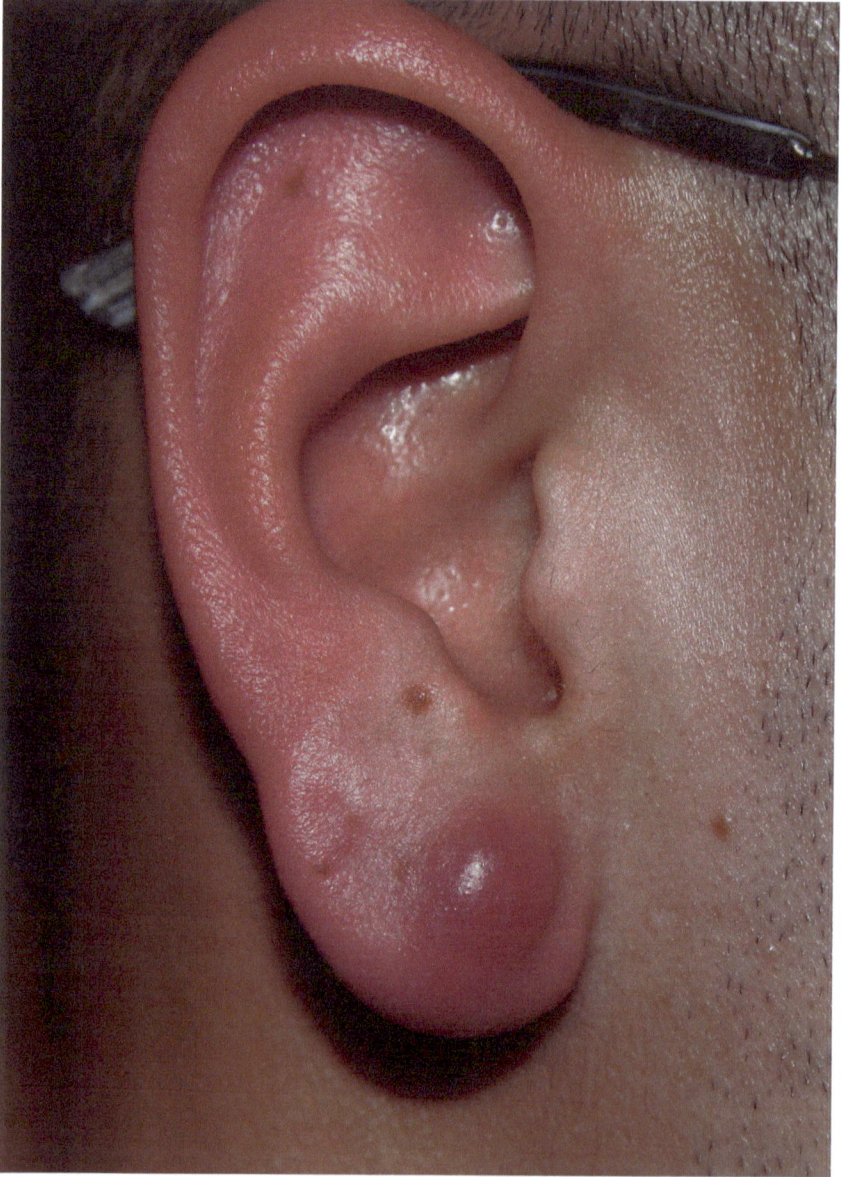

Fig. 26: A small secondary earlobe keloid in a young male.

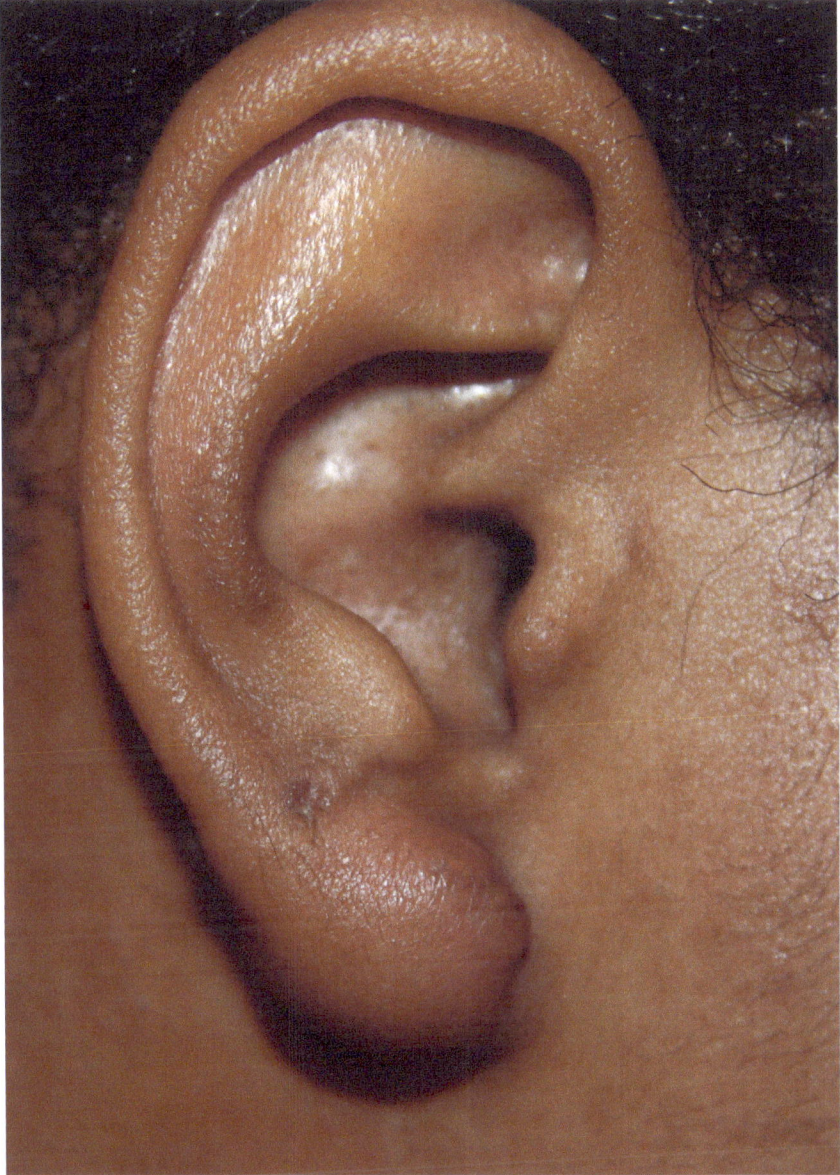

Fig. 27: A secondary earlobe keloid involving the whole thickness of the earlobe.

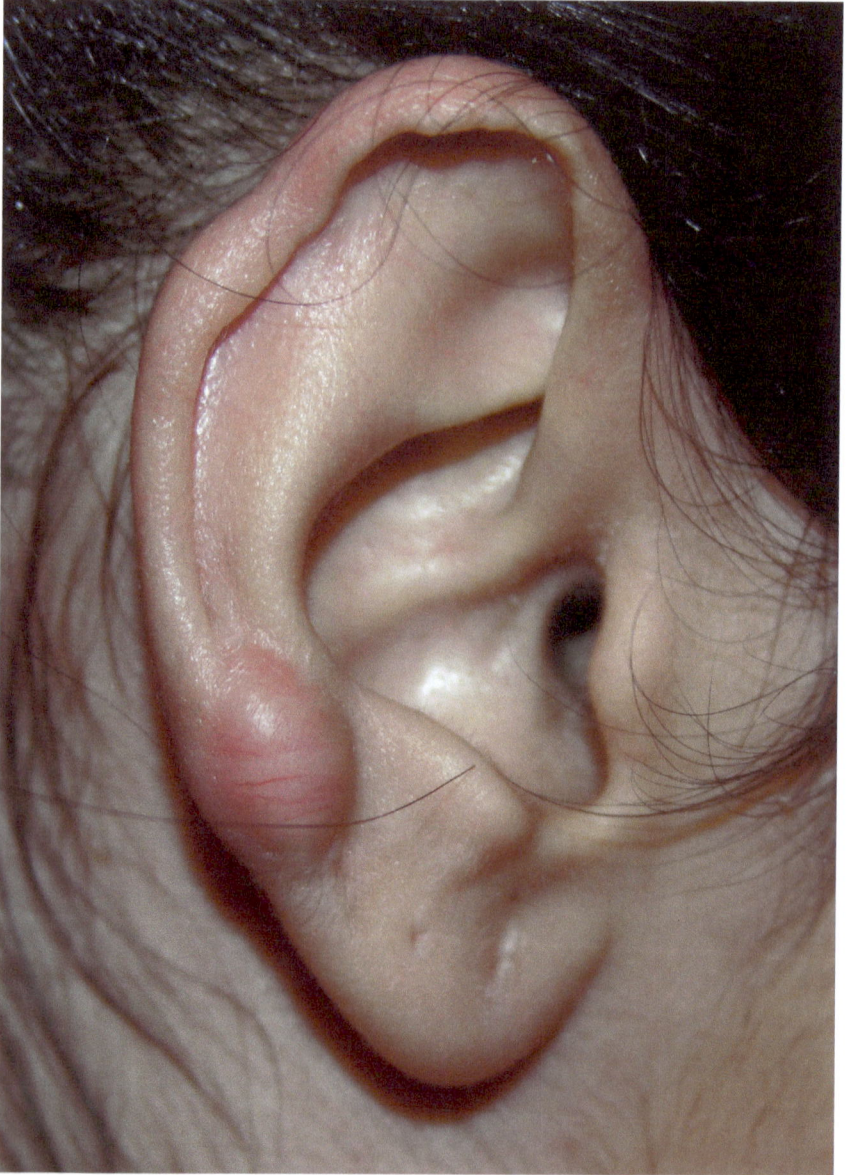

Fig. 28: A small secondary earlobe keloid in a young female. Notice that she did not develop keloids at two other piercing sites.

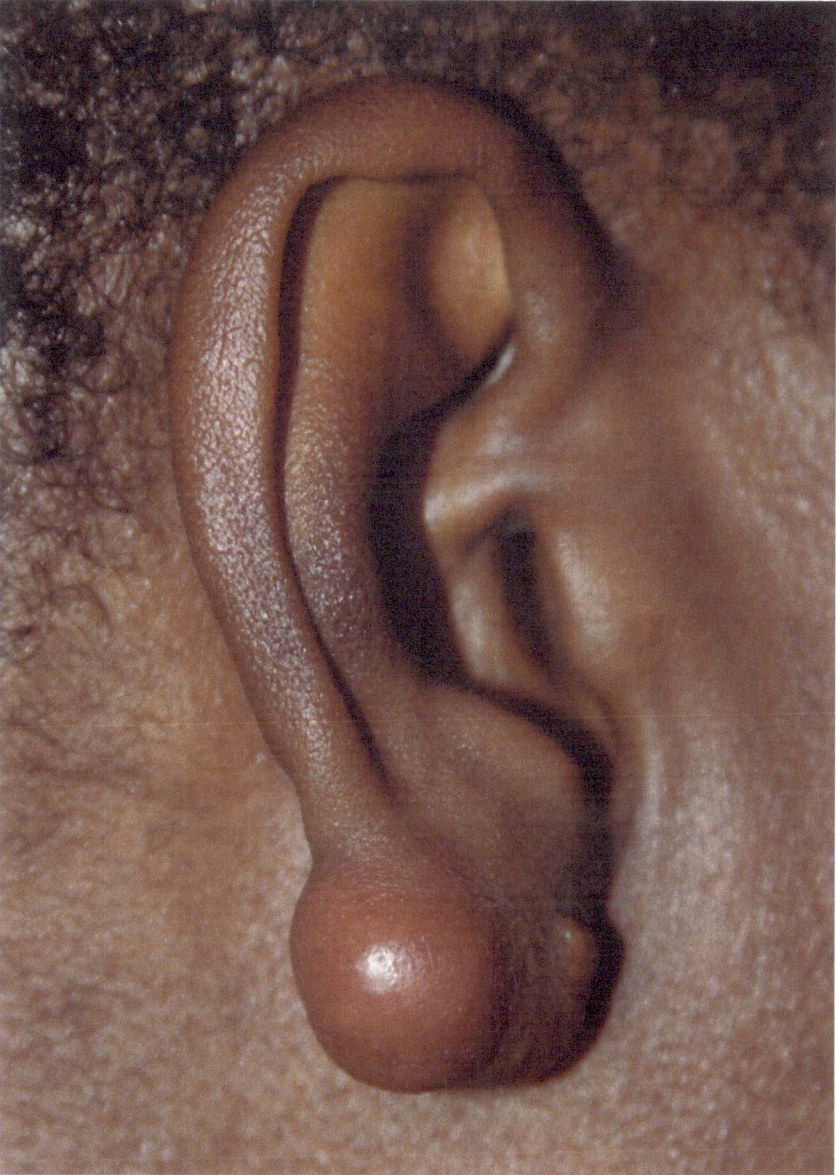

Fig. 29: A medium size secondary earlobe keloid involving much of the earlobe.

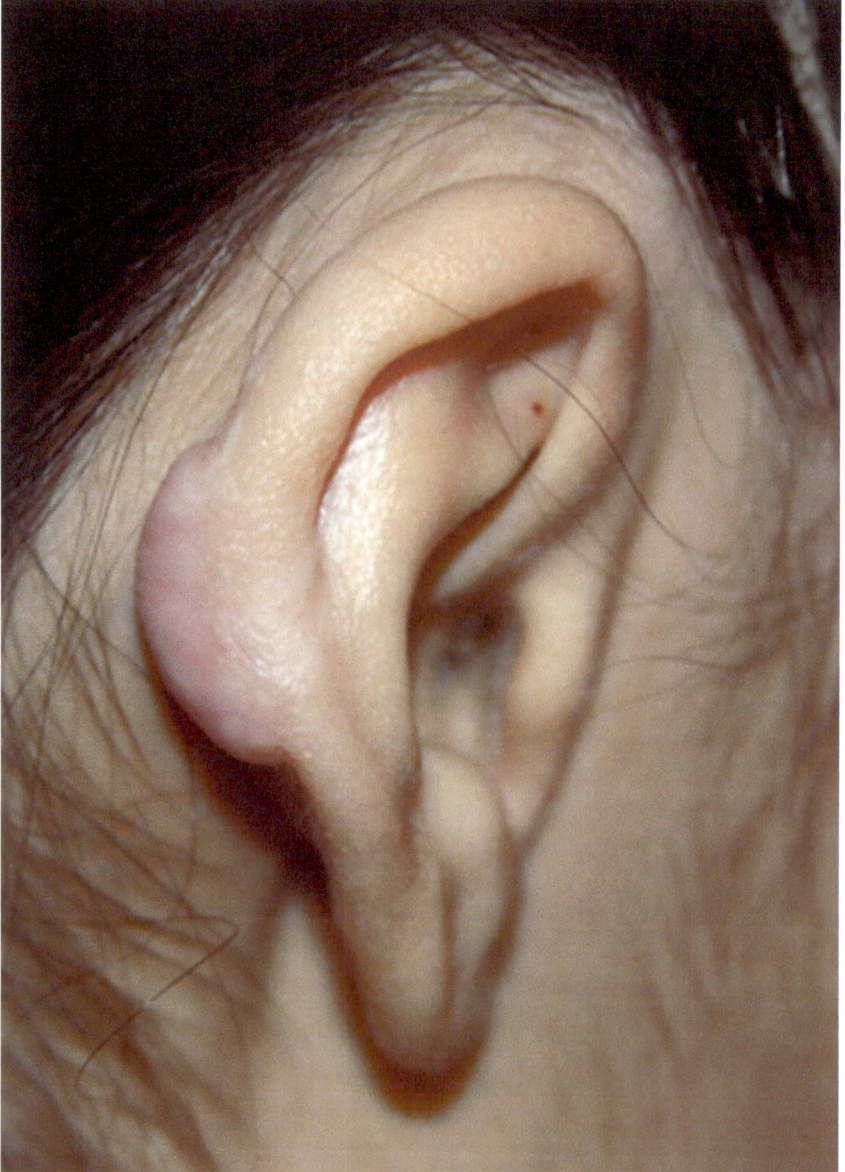

Fig. 30: A secondary ear keloid growing in the posterior surface of the helix.

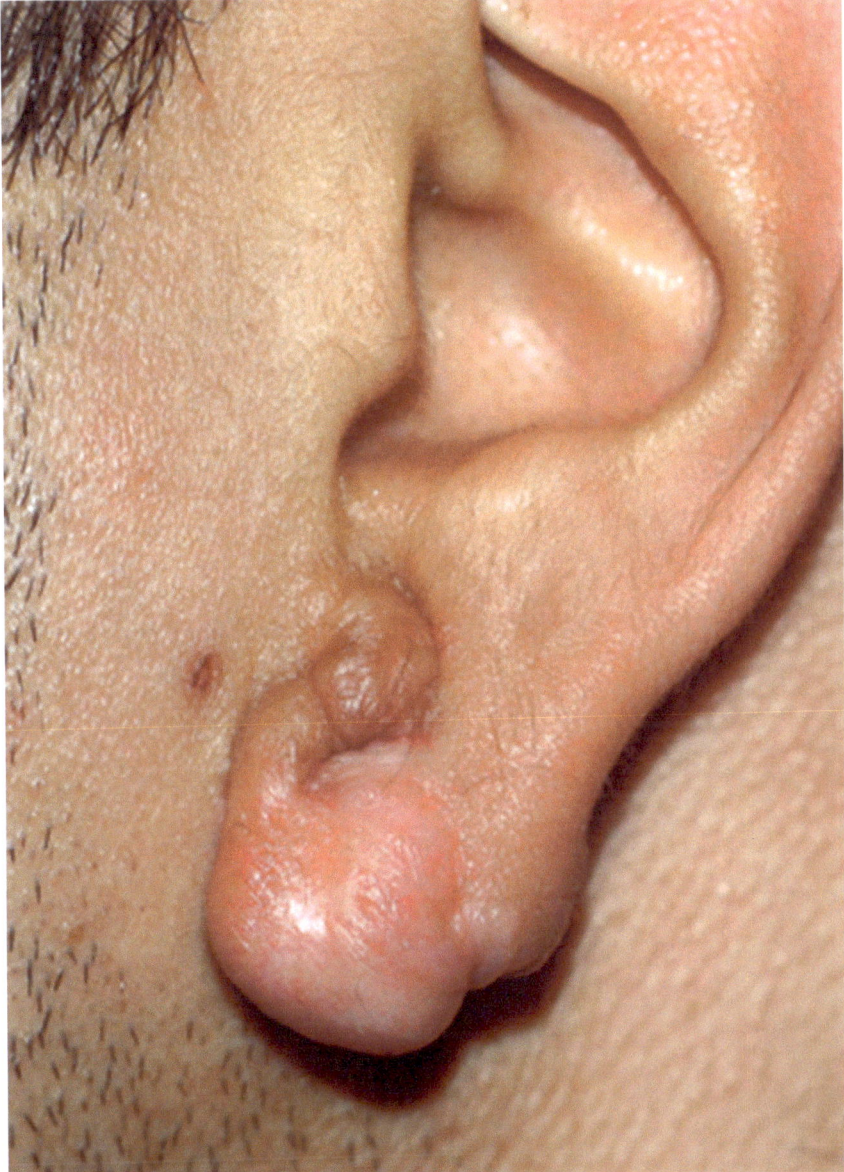

Fig. 31: Recurrence of keloid leading to disfigurement of earlobe.

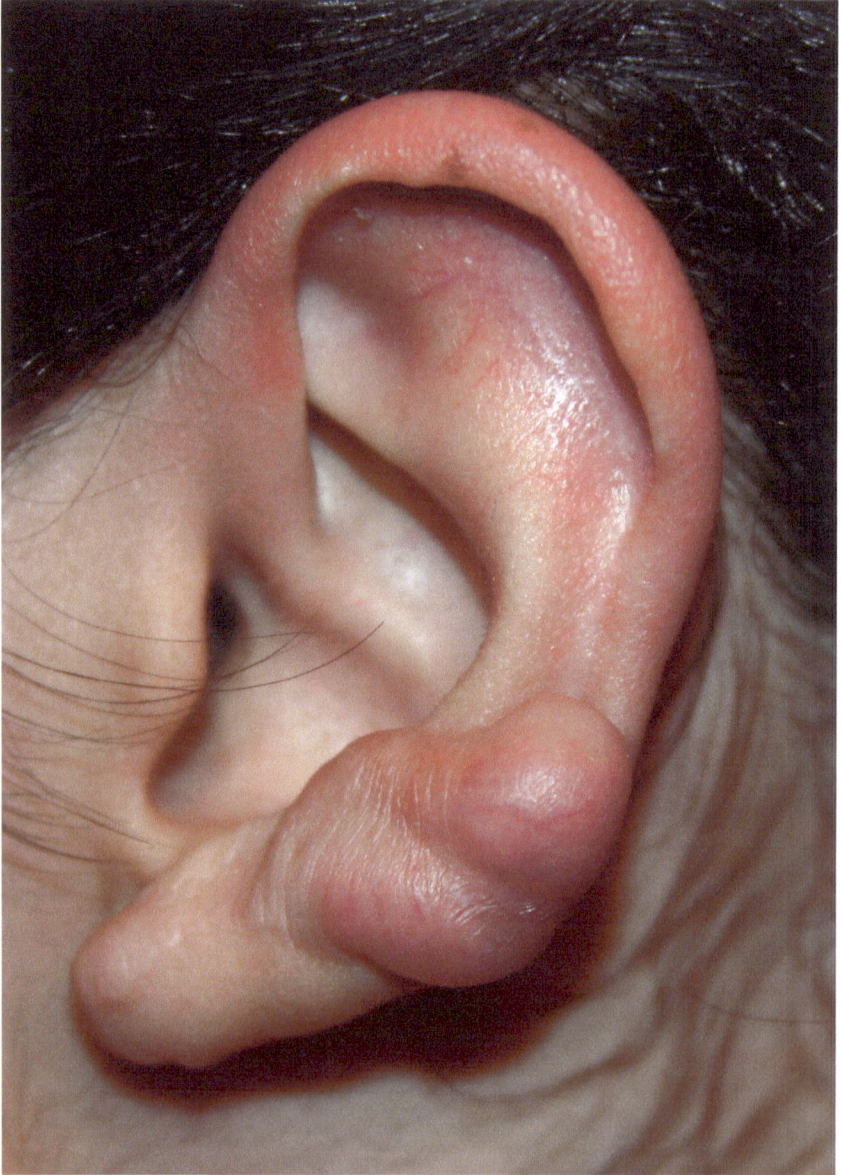

Fig. 32: Recurrence of keloid leading to disfigurement of ear associated with partial disfigurement of the earlobe.

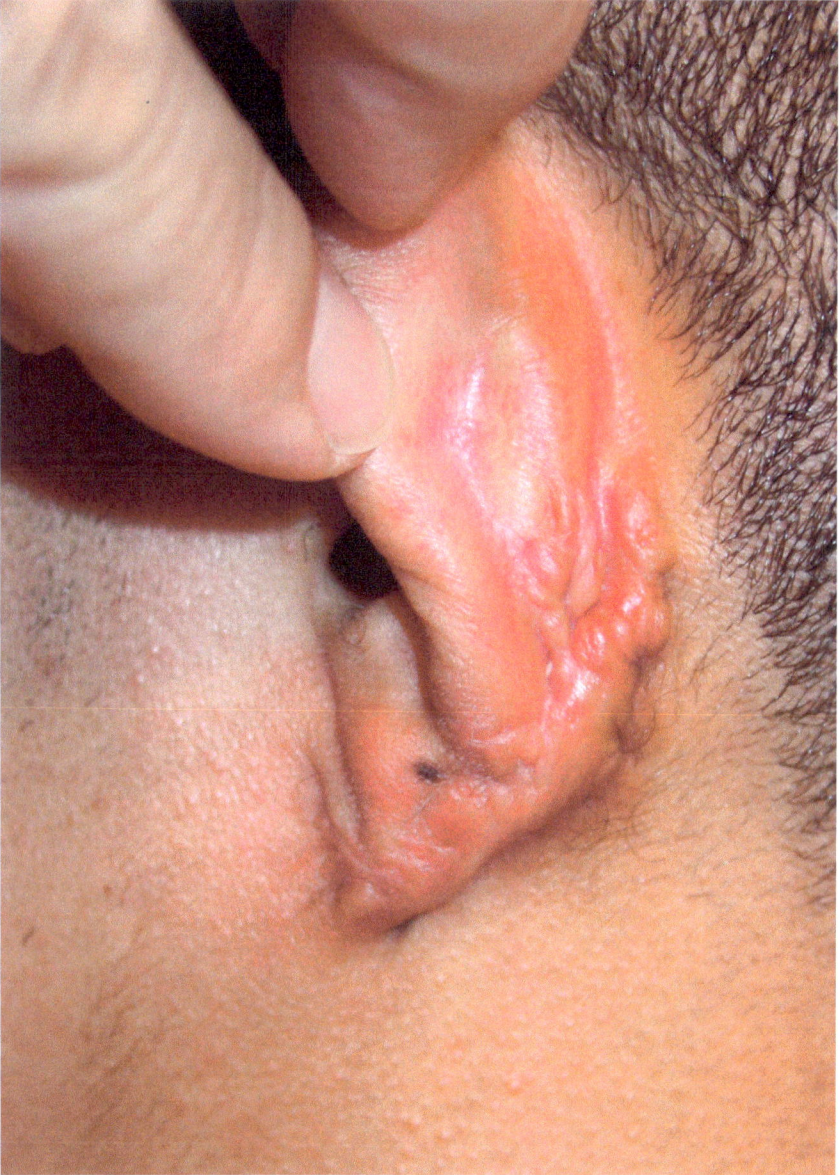

Fig. 33: Recurrence of keloid following total removal of the earlobe.

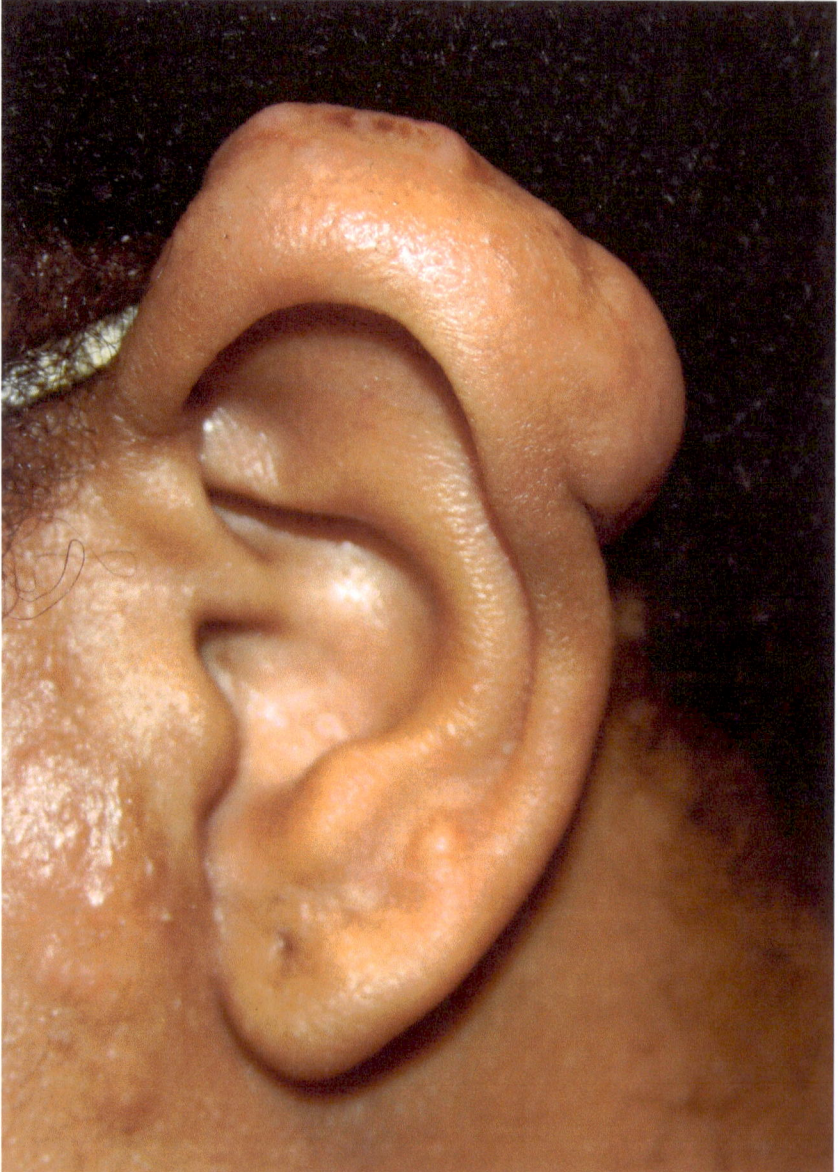

Fig. 34: Large size secondary keloid at the site of surgery to remove a prior helix keloid.

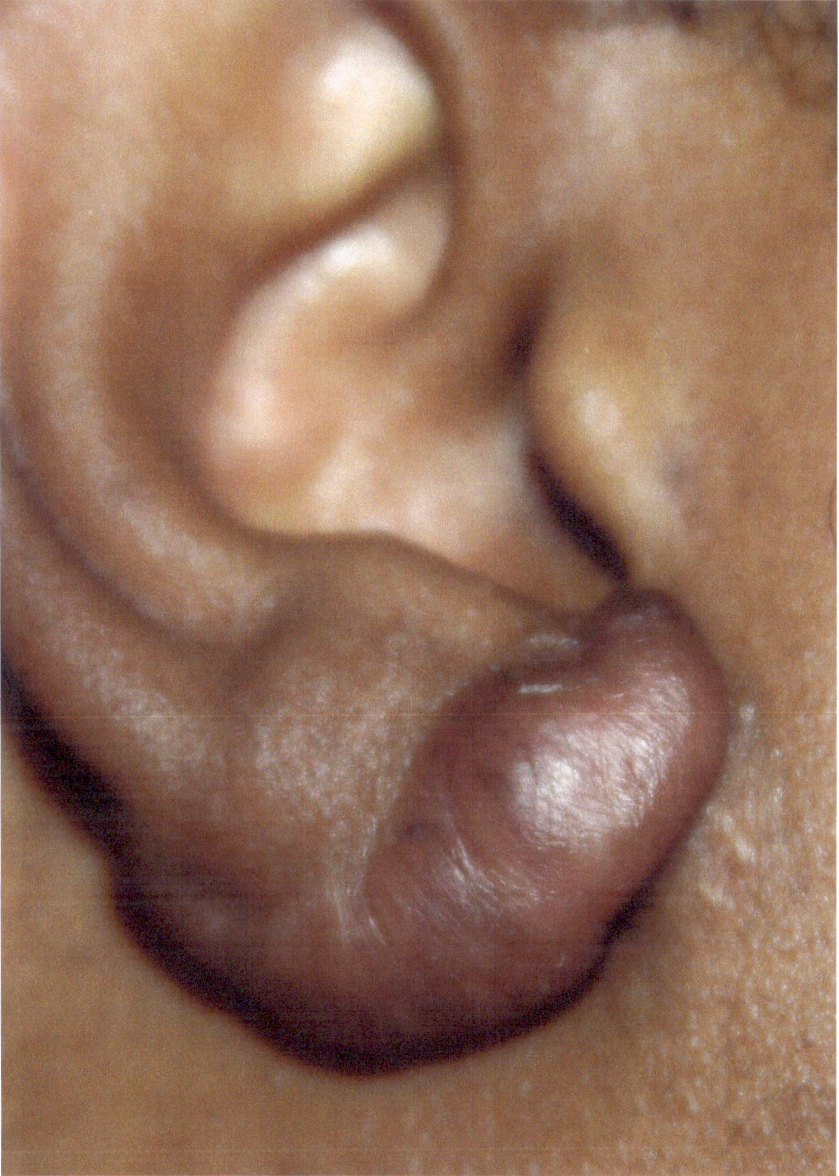

Fig. 35: Recurrence of keloid following total removal of the earlobe.

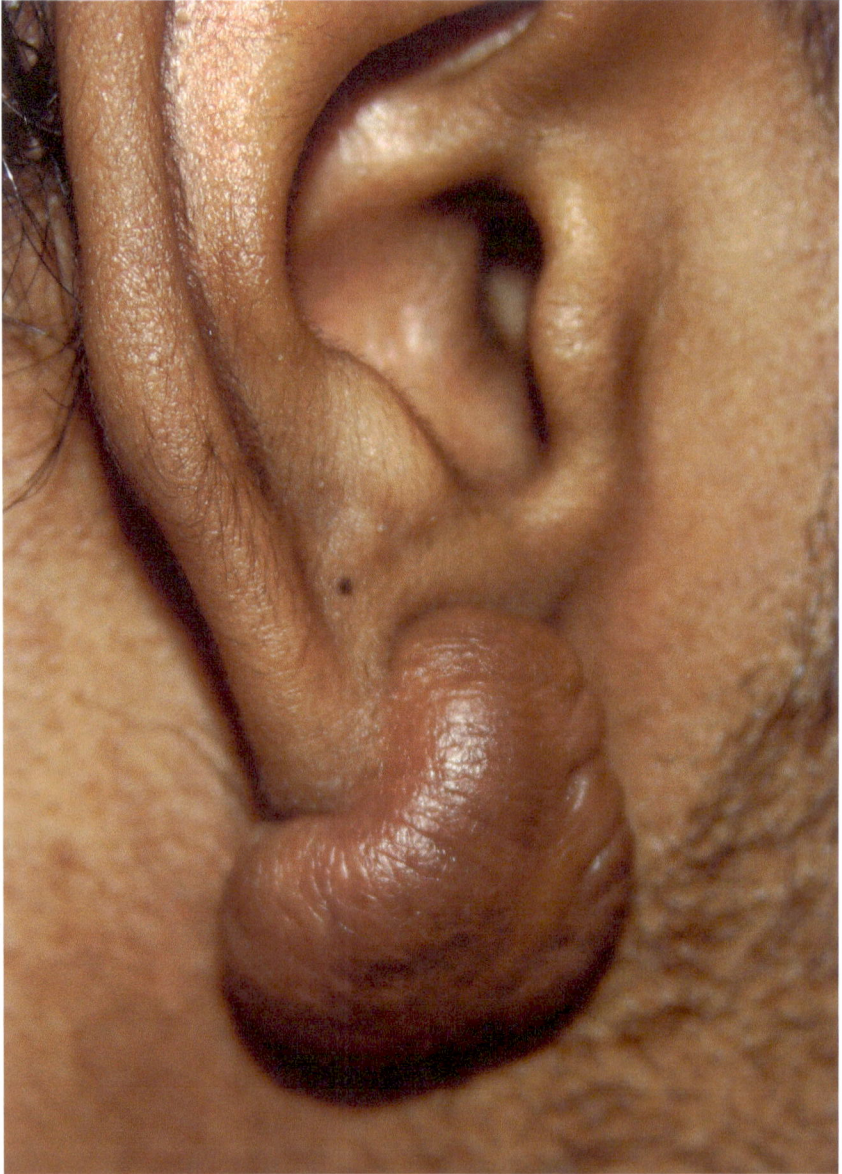

Fig. 36: Recurrence of keloid following total removal of the earlobe.

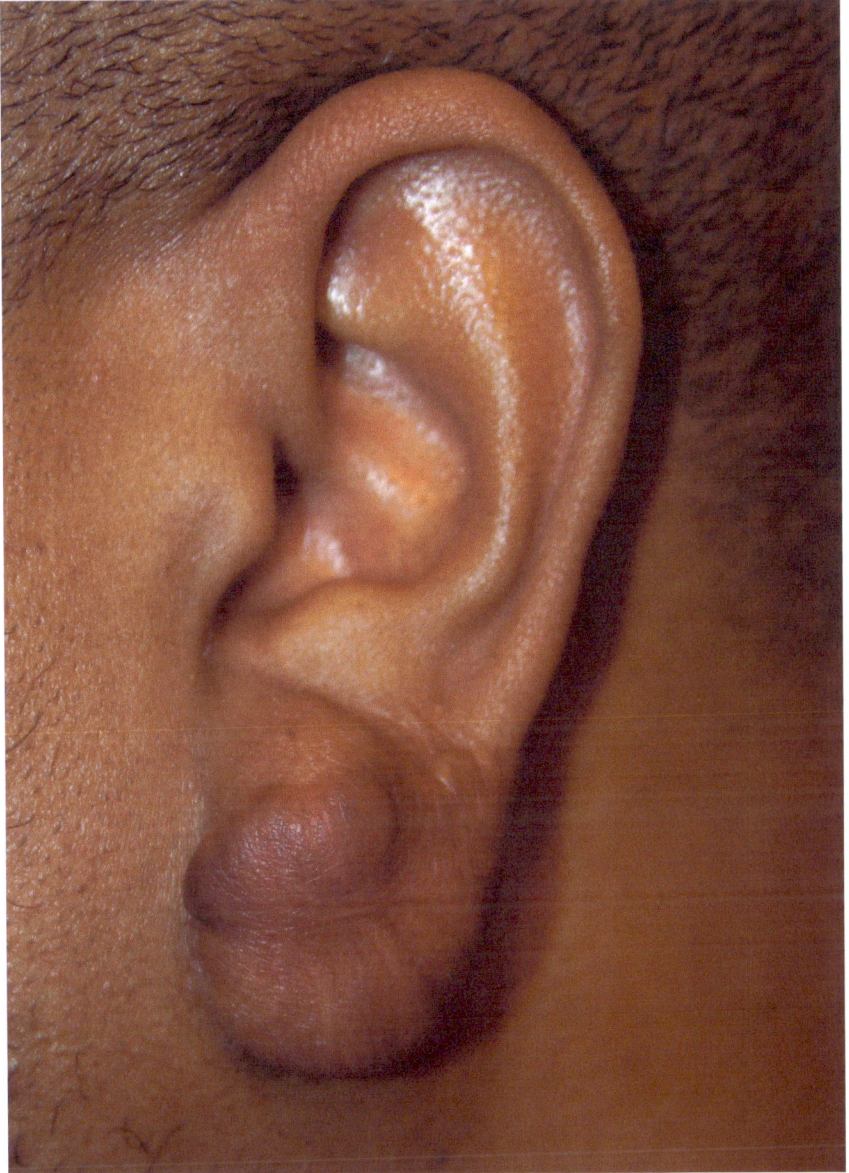

Fig. 37: Recurrence of keloid following partial removal of the earlobe.

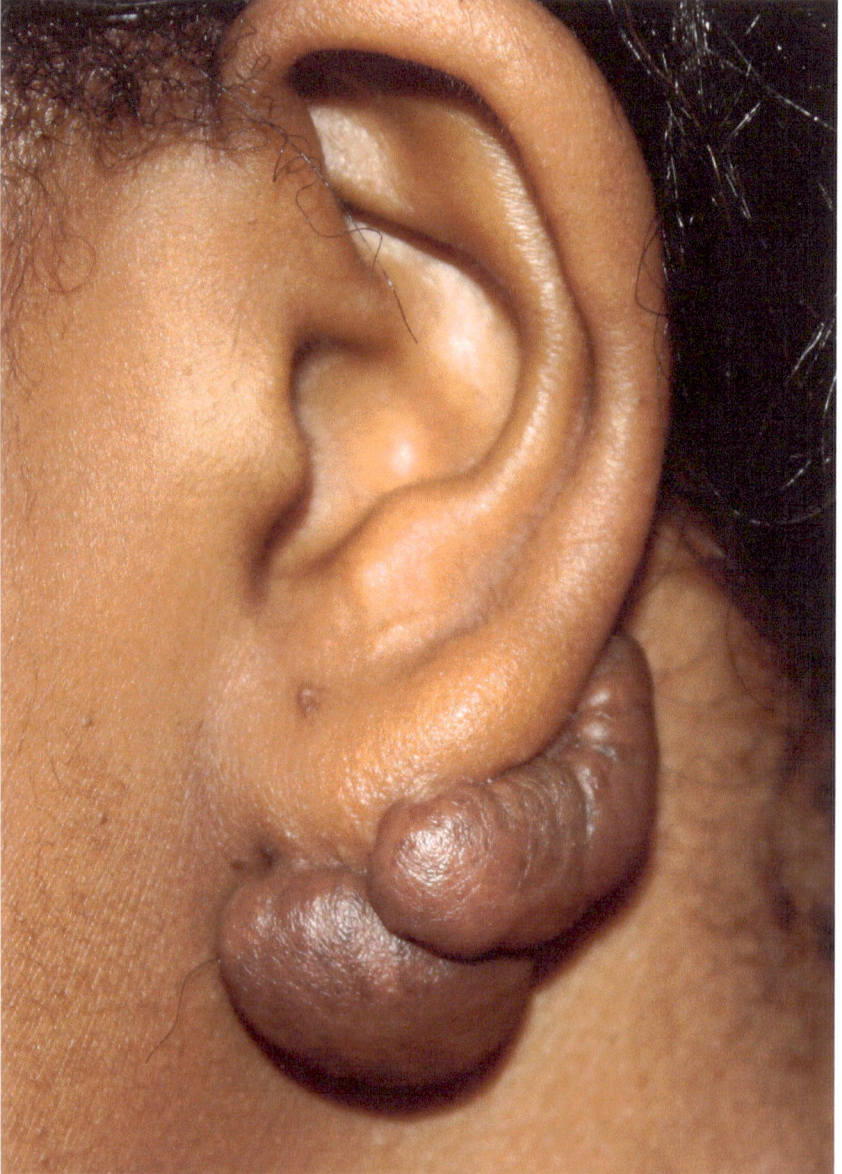

Fig. 38: Recurrence of keloid at the site of surgery for removal of a prior earlobe keloid.

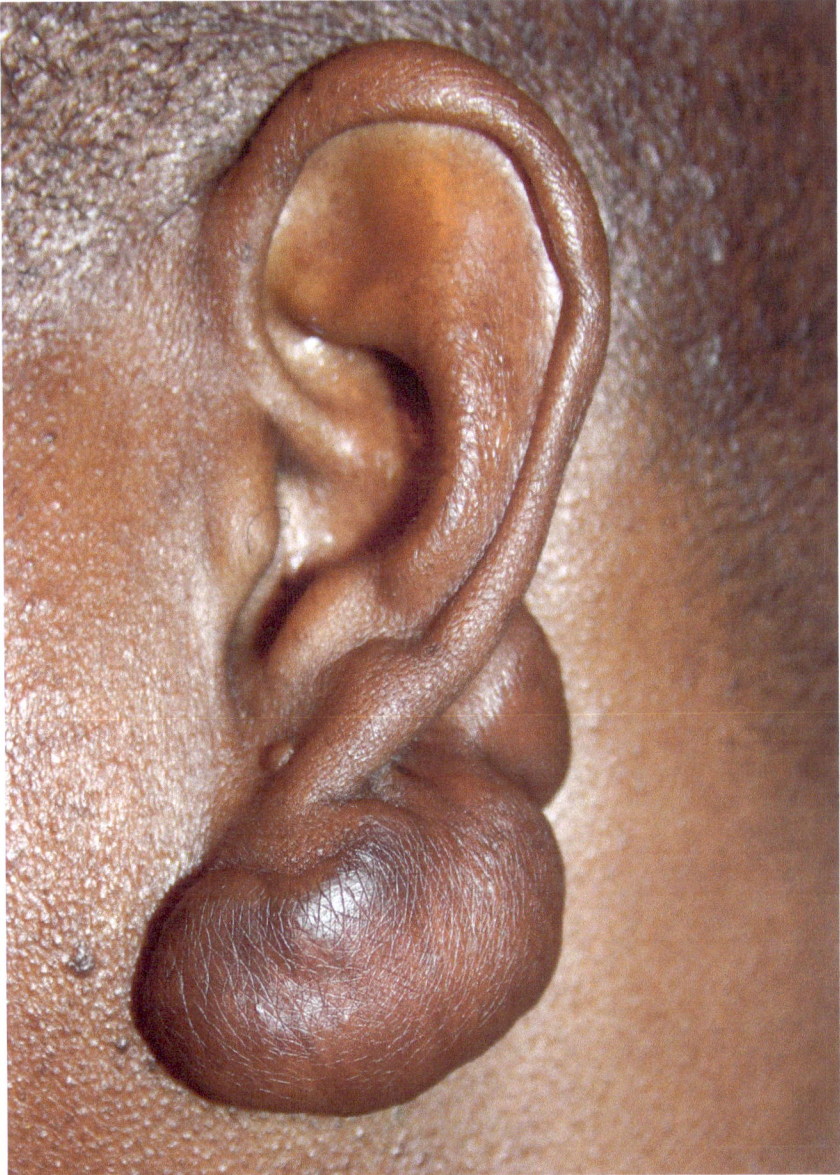

Fig. 39: Complex local recurrence, secondary earlobe keloid.

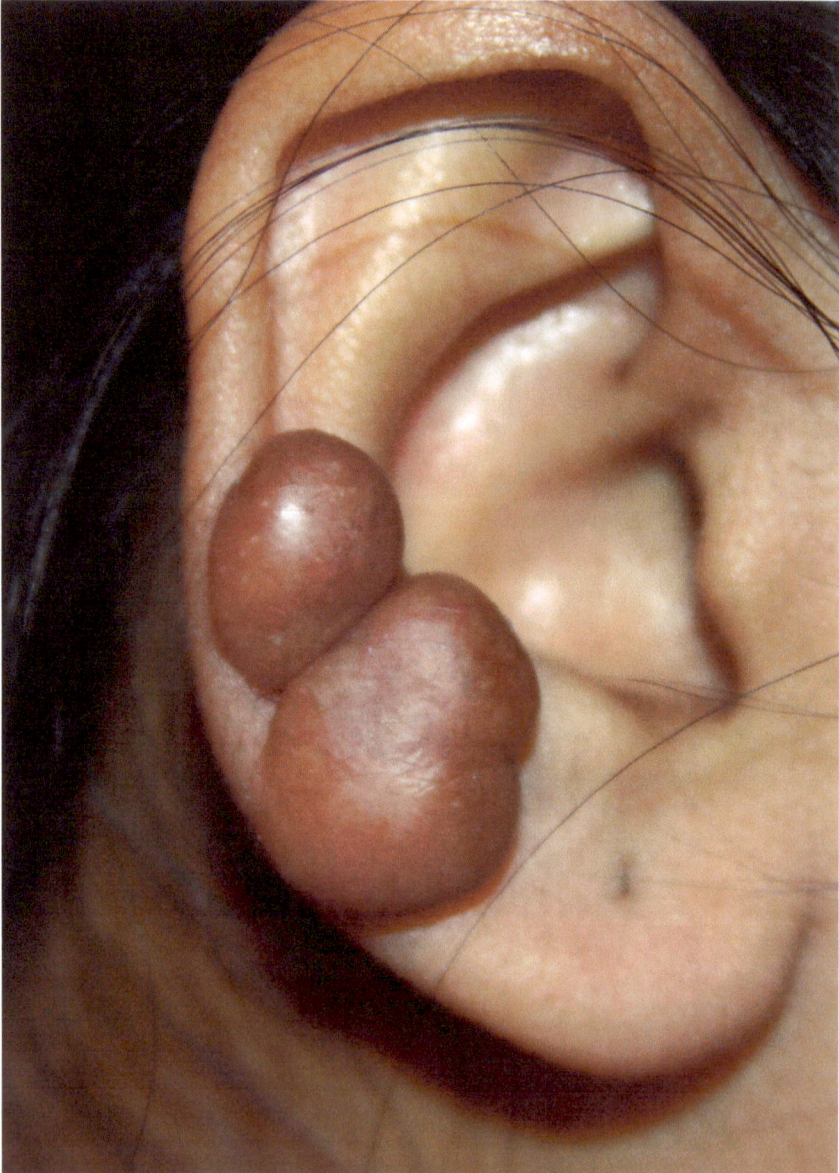

Fig. 40: Recurrence of keloid following the removal of an ear keloid.

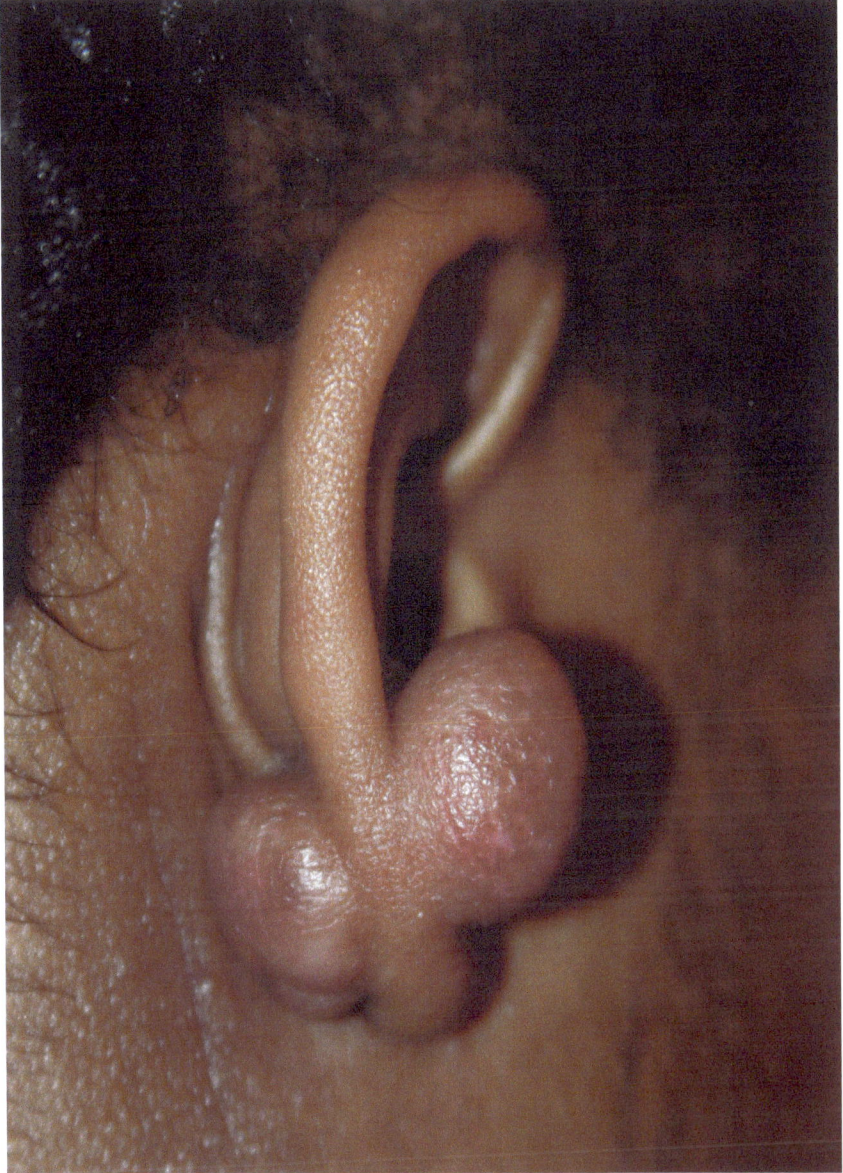

Fig. 41: Recurrence of keloid on both surfaces of the earlobe.

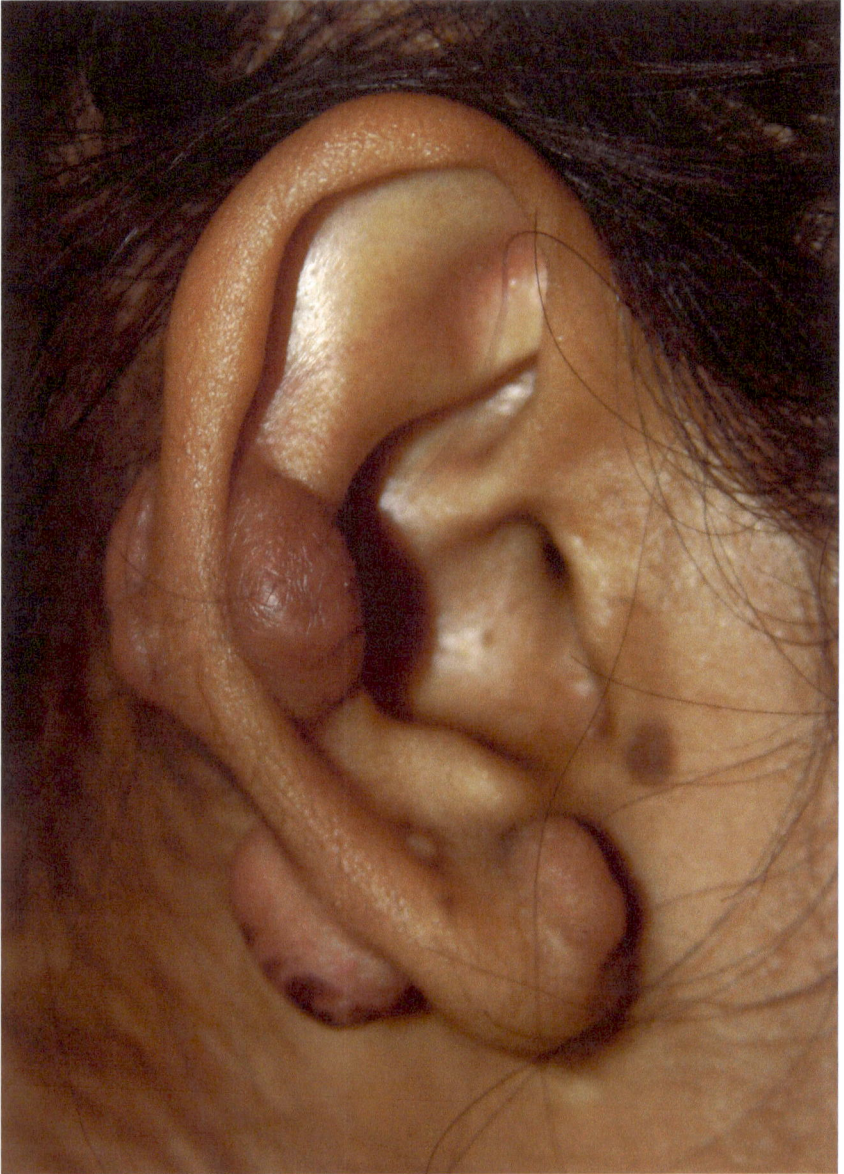

Fig. 42: Recurrence of keloids following surgical removal of multiple ear keloids.

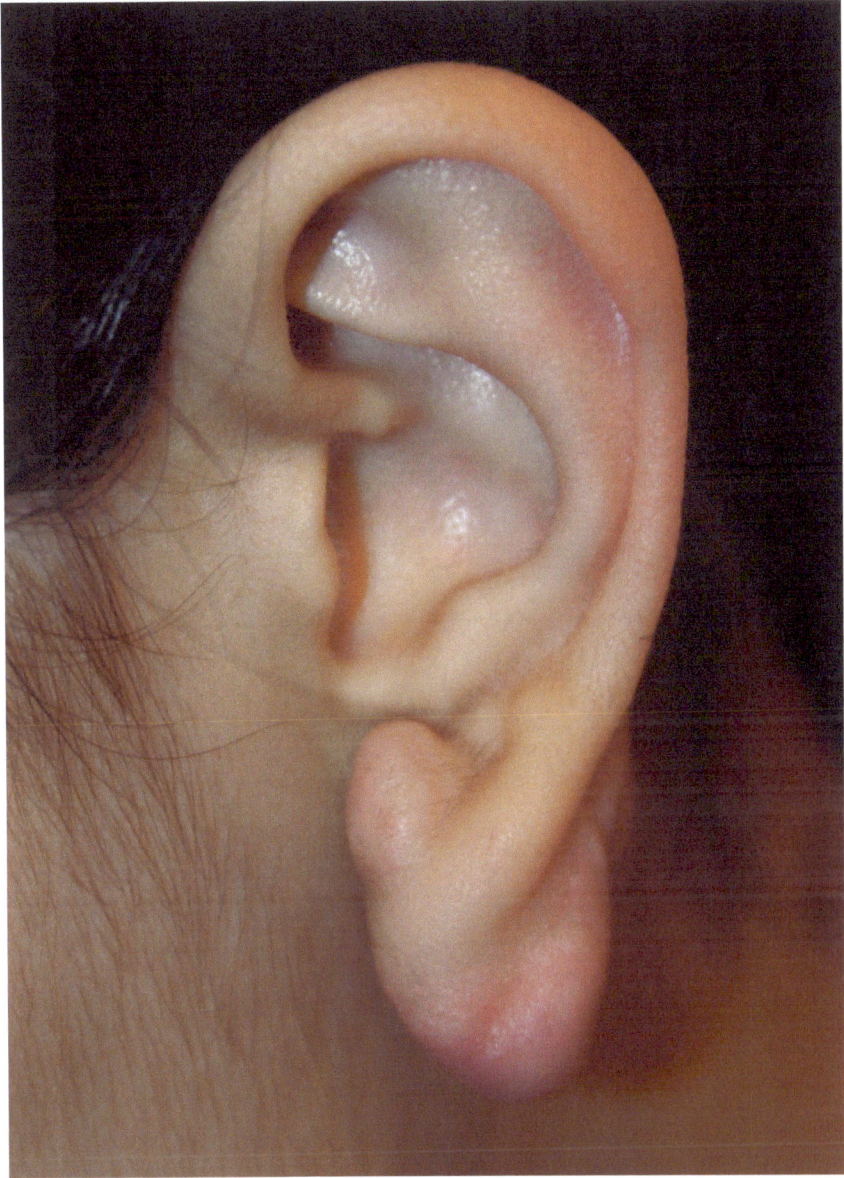

Fig. 43: Recurrence of keloid on both surfaces of the earlobe. Note that keloids are of different size and shape.

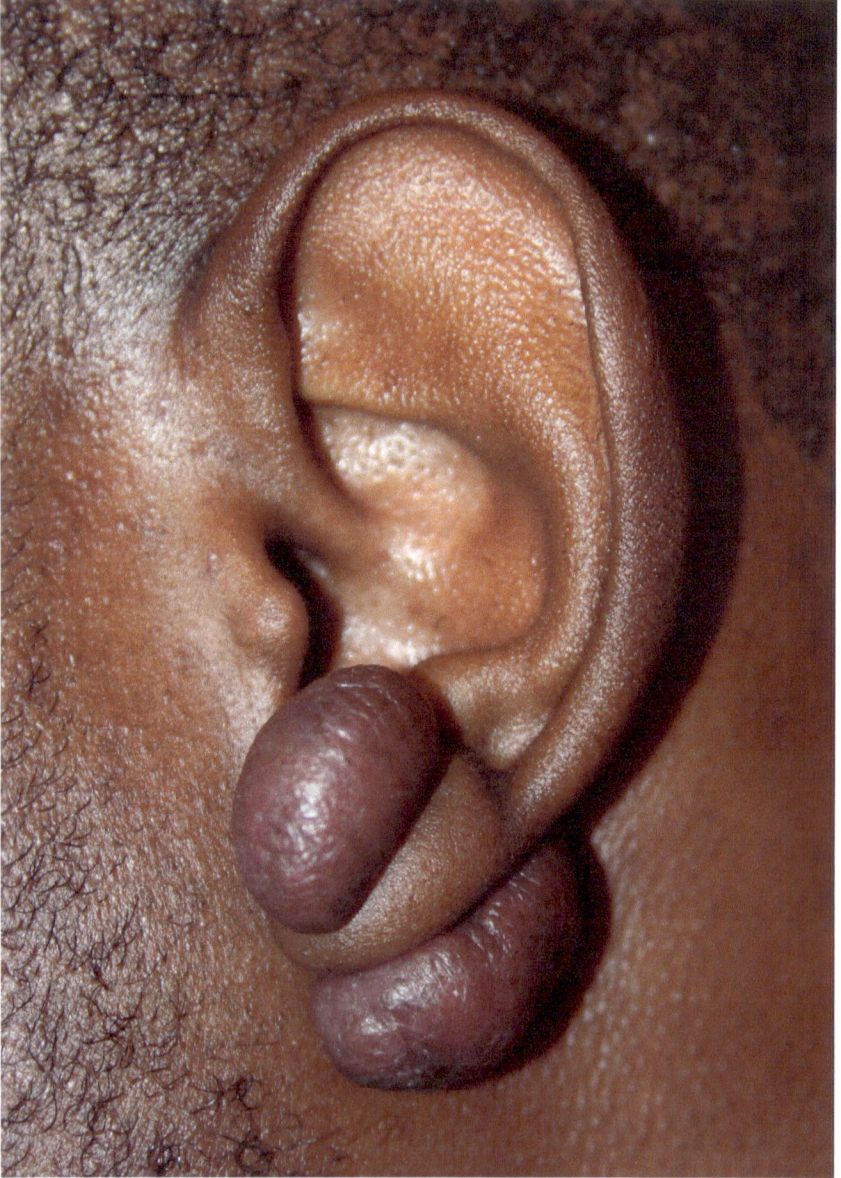

Fig. 44: Recurrence of keloid following removal of earlobe keloids from both surfaces. Note both keloids are almost the same size and maintain the same contour.

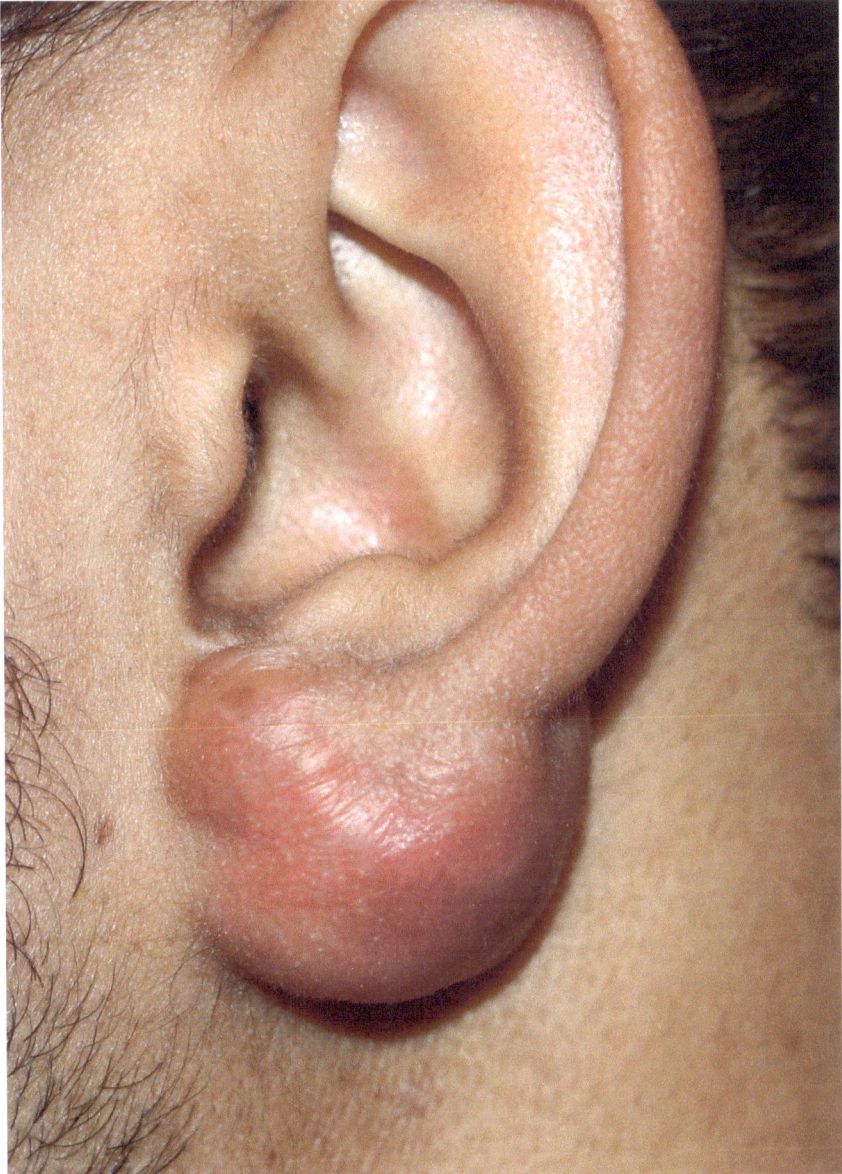

Fig. 45: Keloid tumor formation at the site of recurrence following total removal of the earlobe.

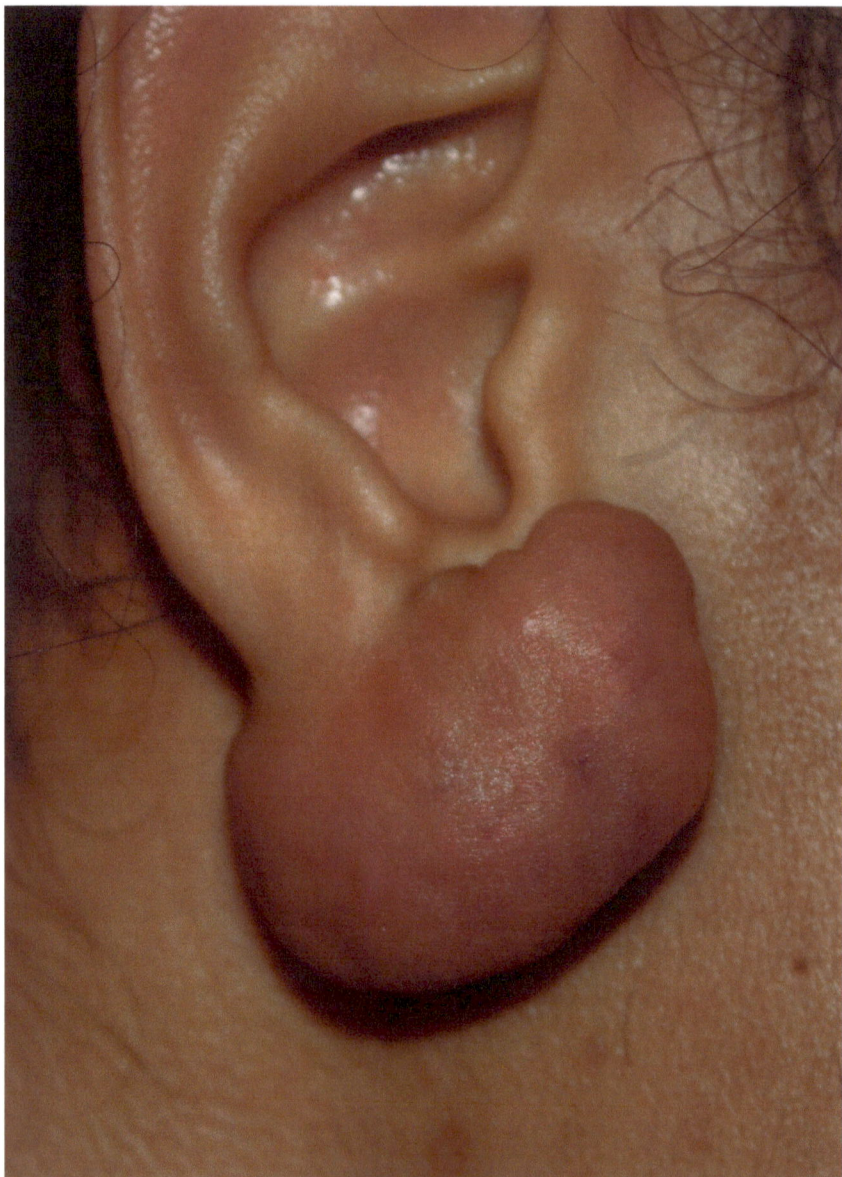

Fig. 46: A more advanced case of recurrent keloid. Note the total destruction of the earlobe, which is in part due to surgery, and in part due to keloid recurrence.

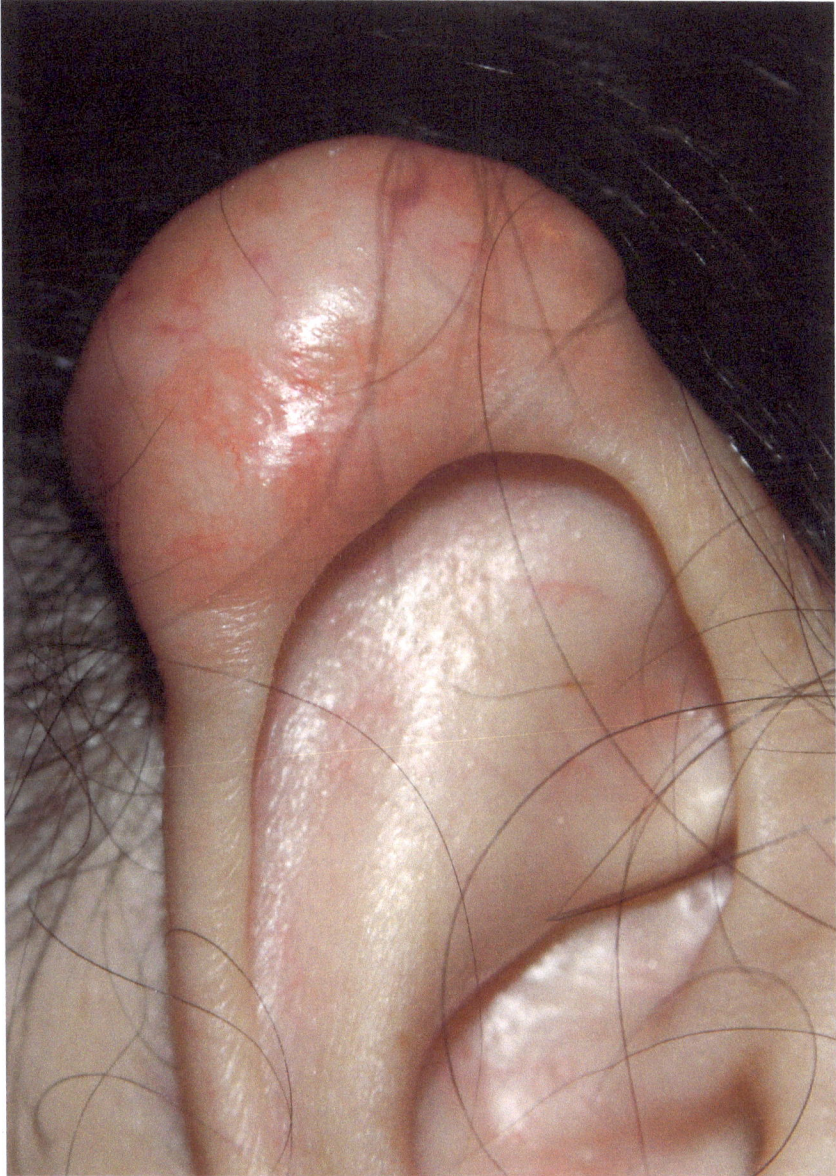

Fig. 47: Disfiguring recurrence of keloid in the helix of the ear. This keloid has been resistant to prior surgeries as well as steroids. Like many other women with similar issues, this patient always kept her hair down, or wore a hat in order to conceal the unsightly appearance of her keloid.

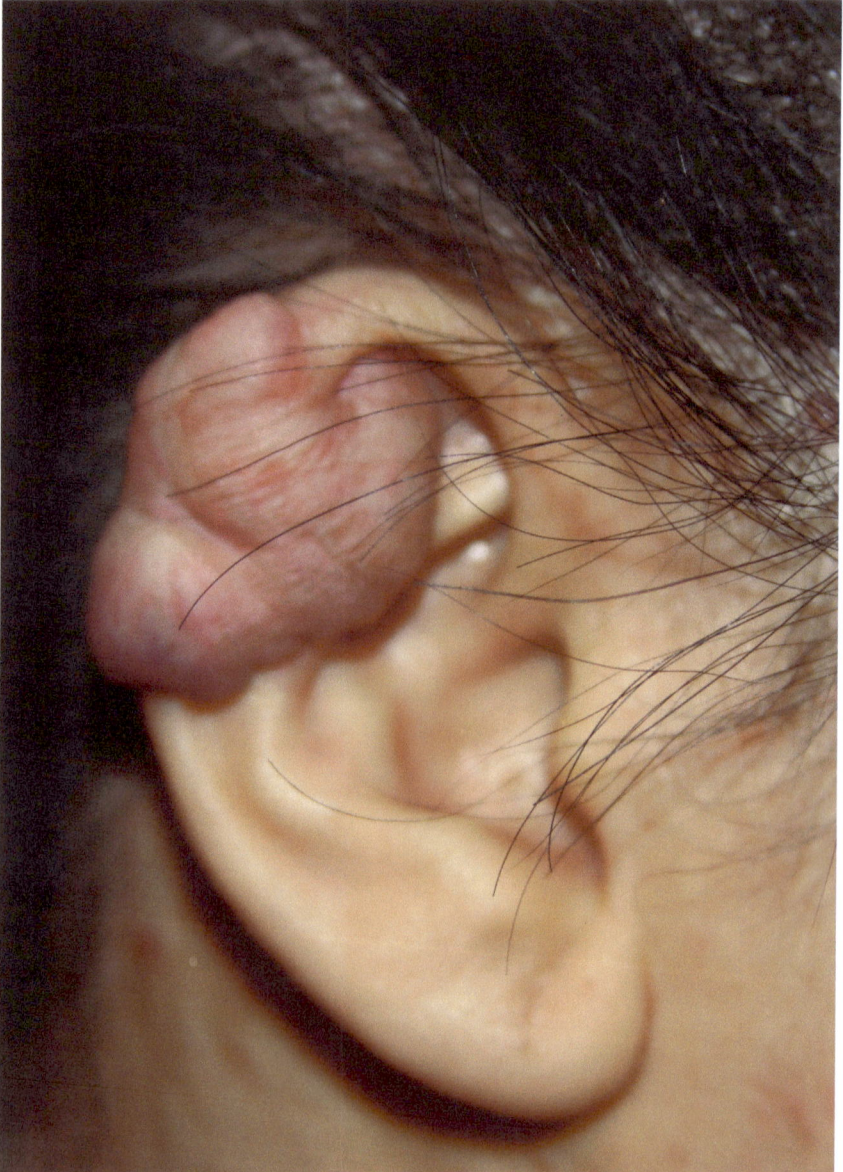

Fig. 48: Disfiguring recurrence of a keloid in the helix of the ear after a wedge resection of a small primary keloid of the helix.

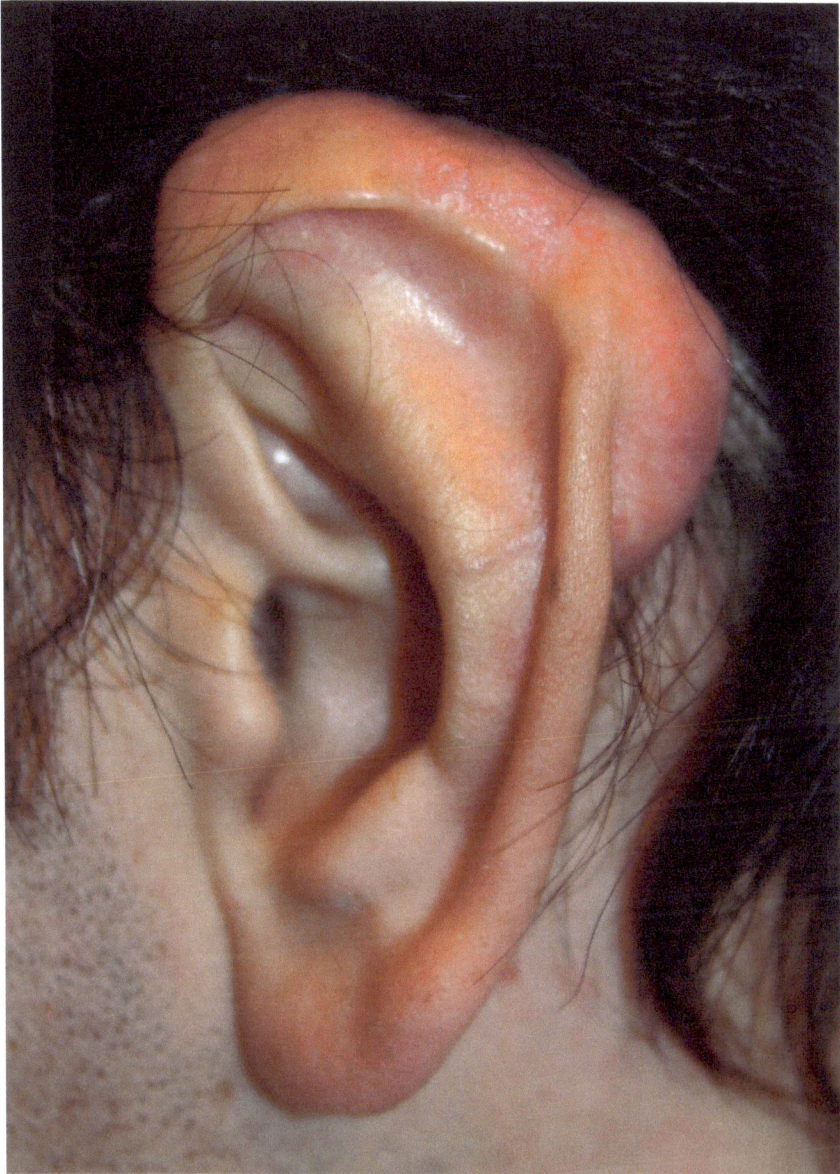

Fig. 49: Disfiguring and large recurrence of keloid in the helix of the ear after multiple wedge resection surgeries for a small primary keloid of the helix.

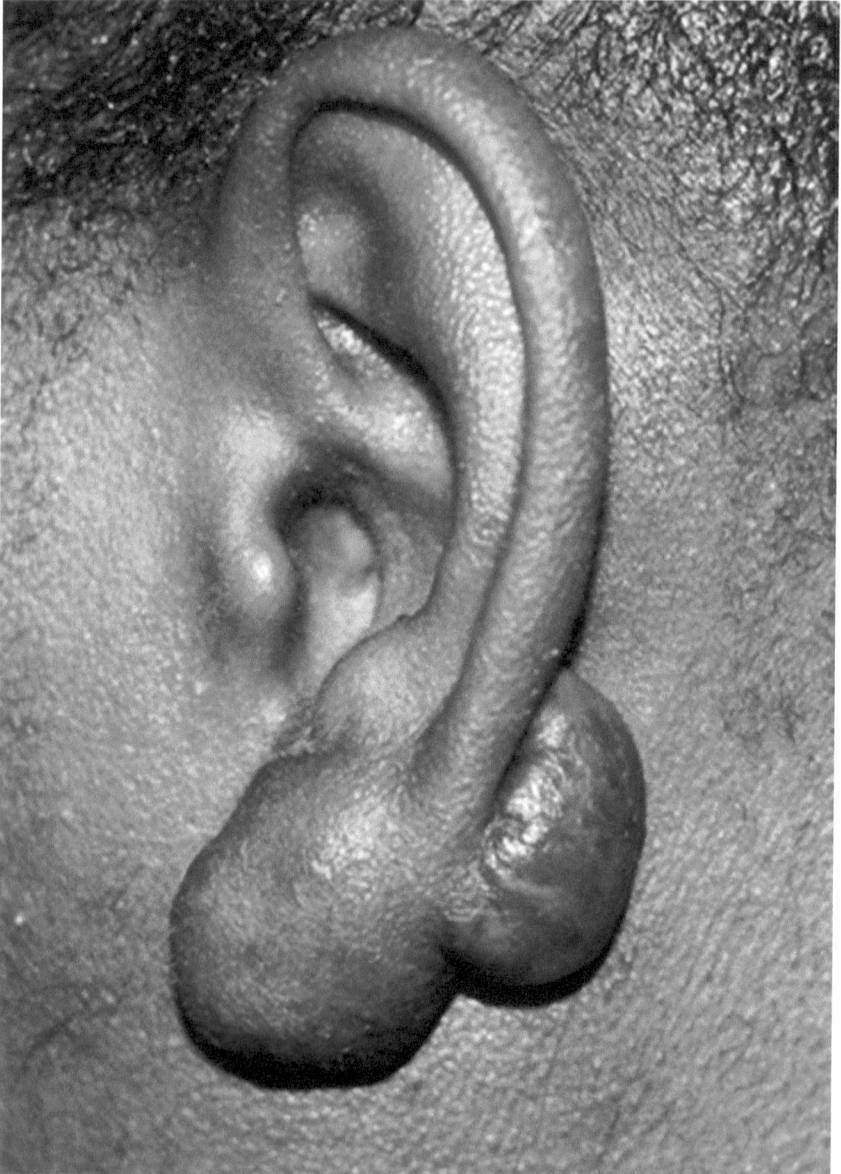

Fig. 50: Fifteen year-old female who has undergone three surgeries as well as radiation therapy. Her earlobe keloid and the appearance of her left ear is considerably worse than ever before.

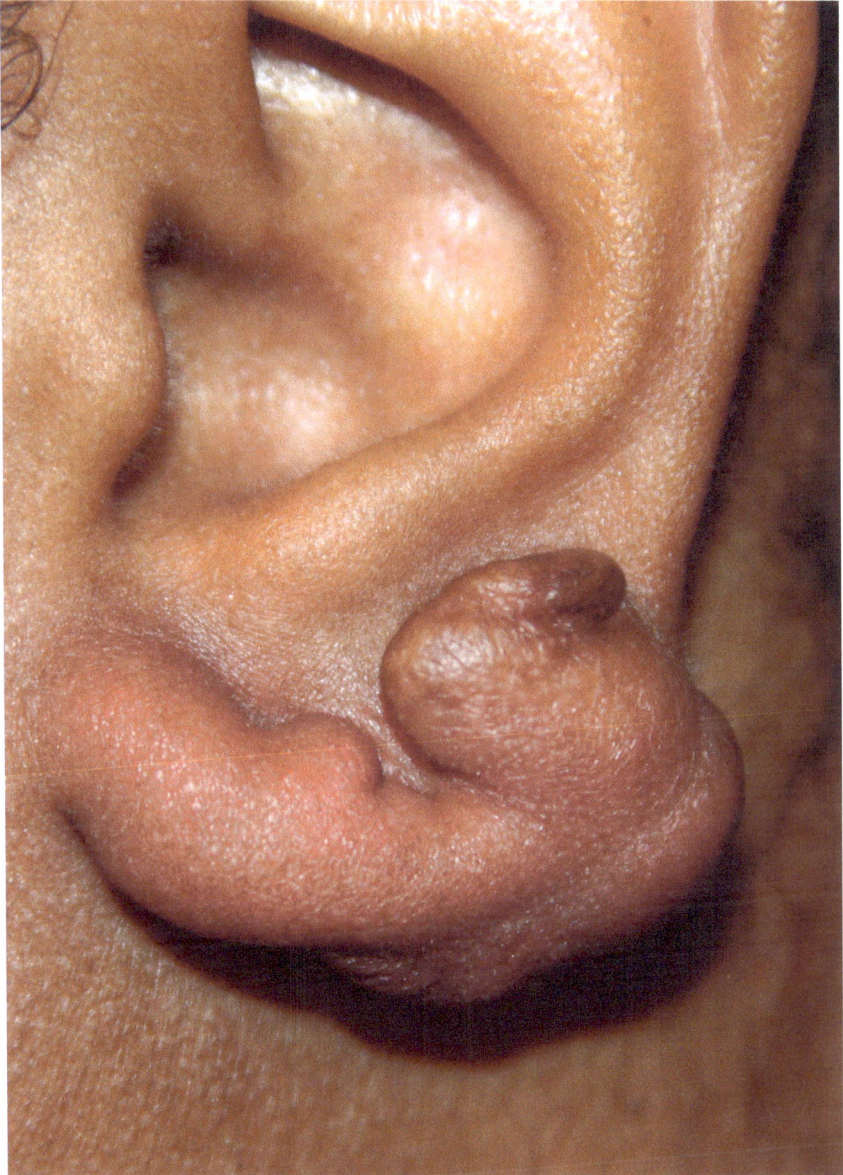

Fig. 51: Disfiguring and complex recurrence of an earlobe keloid.

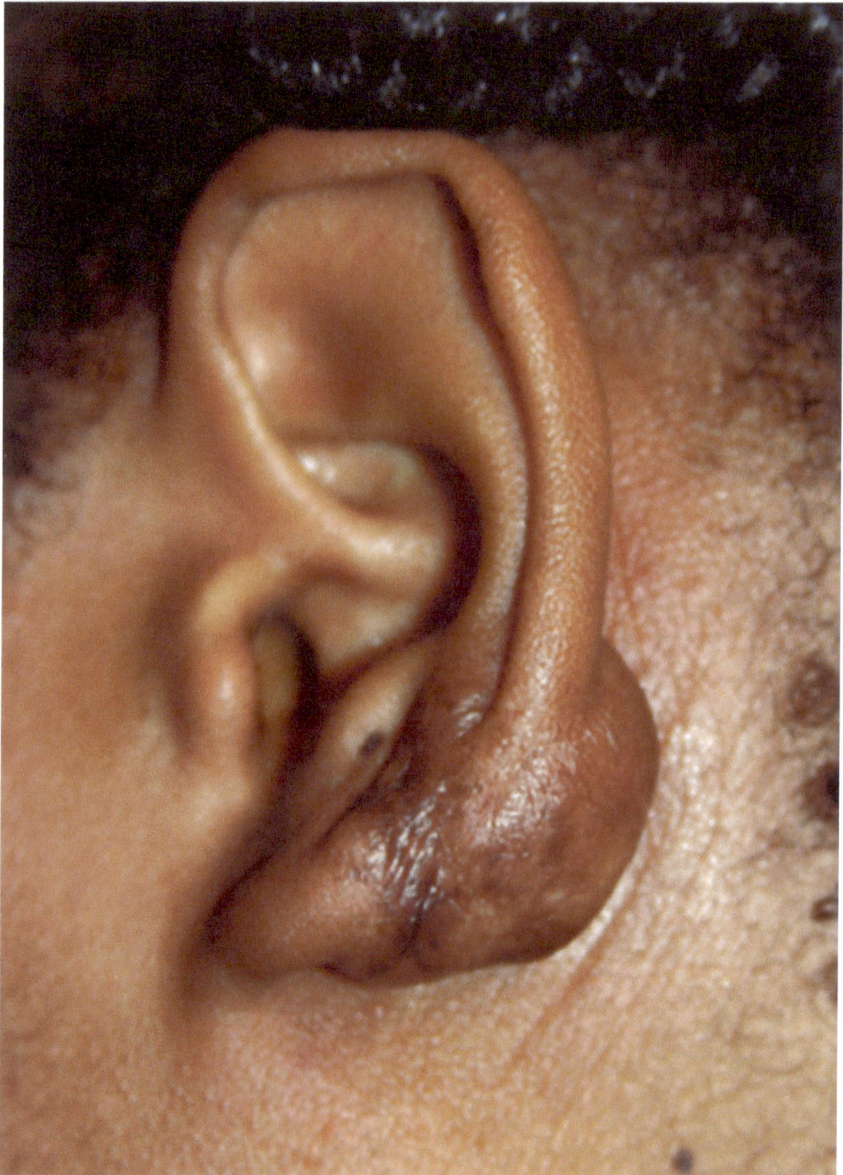

Fig. 52: Disfiguring and large recurrence of keloid above the earlobe after a wedge resection surgery.

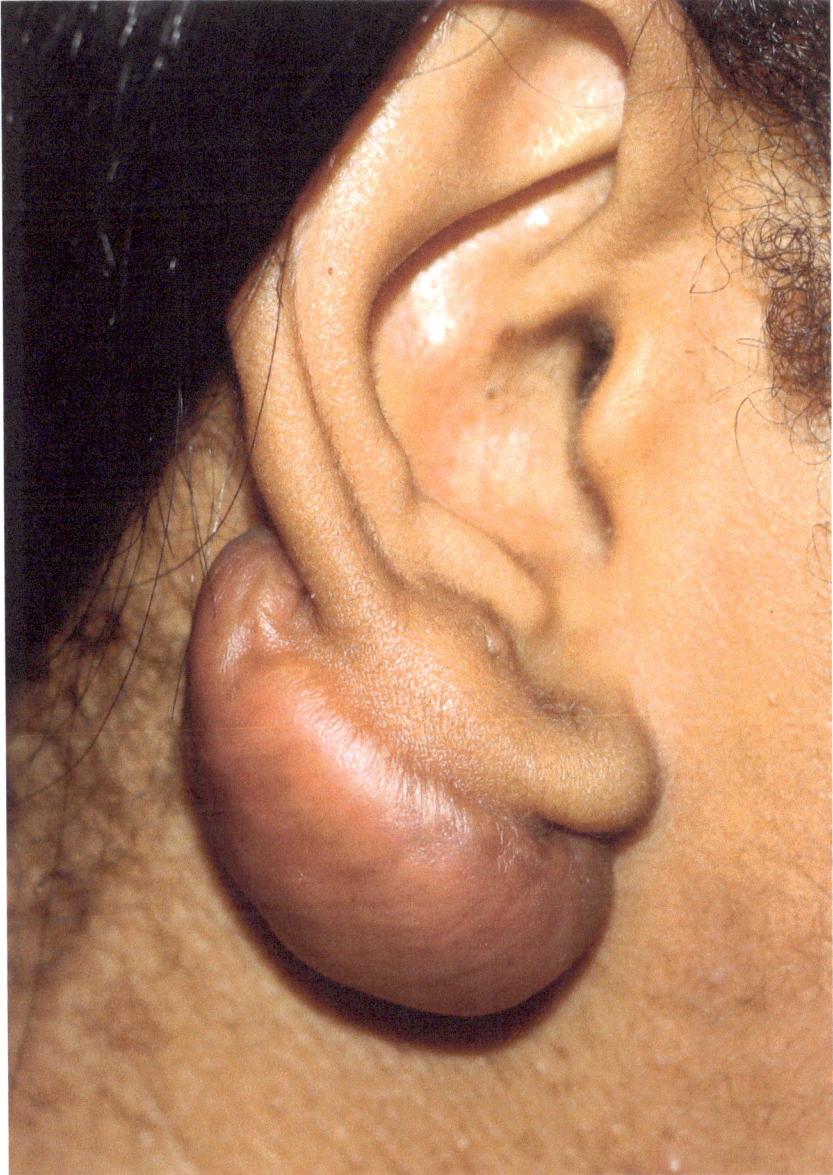

Fig. 53: Disfiguring and large recurrence of a keloid in posterior surface of the right ear.

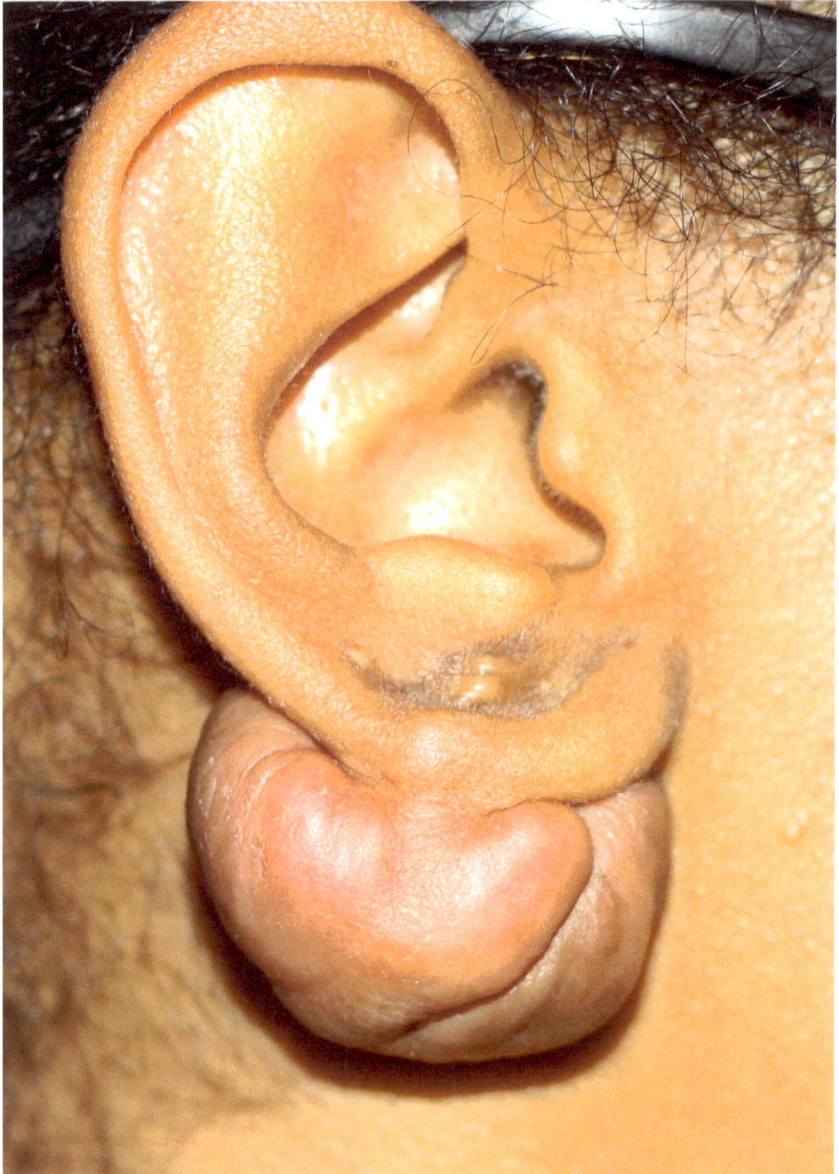

Fig. 54: Disfiguring, large and complex recurrence of earlobe keloid.

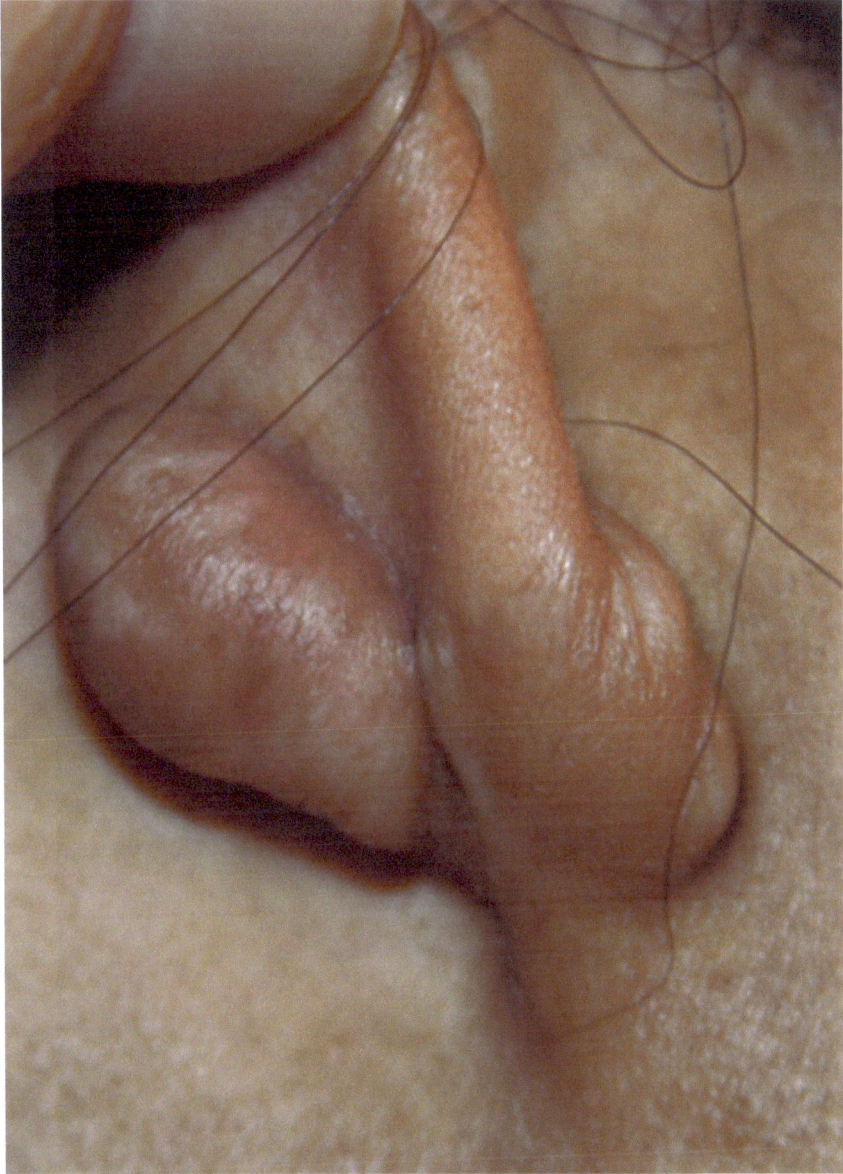

Fig. 55: Recurrence of a keloid after total resection of the earlobe with keloid growth way beyond the surgical wound over mastoid bone.

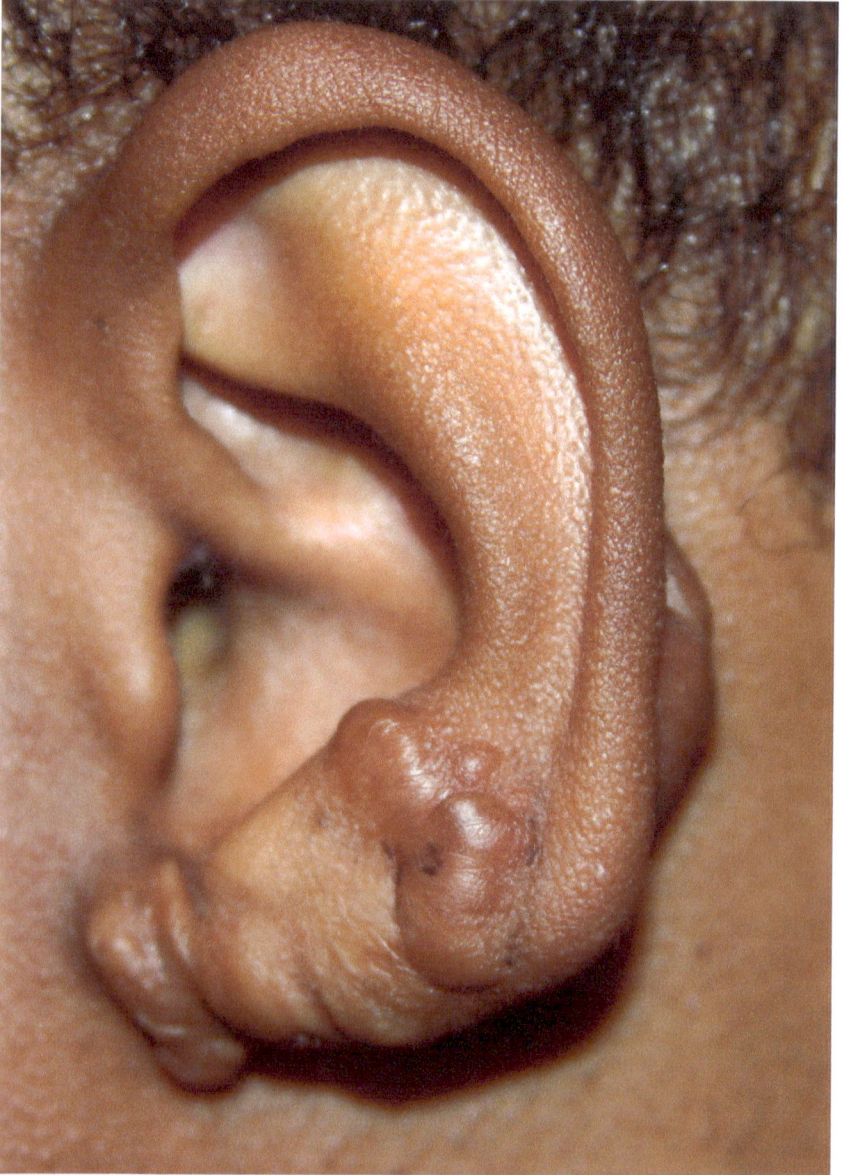

Fig. 56: Recurrence of keloid after multiple surgeries. Notice keloid regrowth on every surgical wound as well as behind the earlobe.

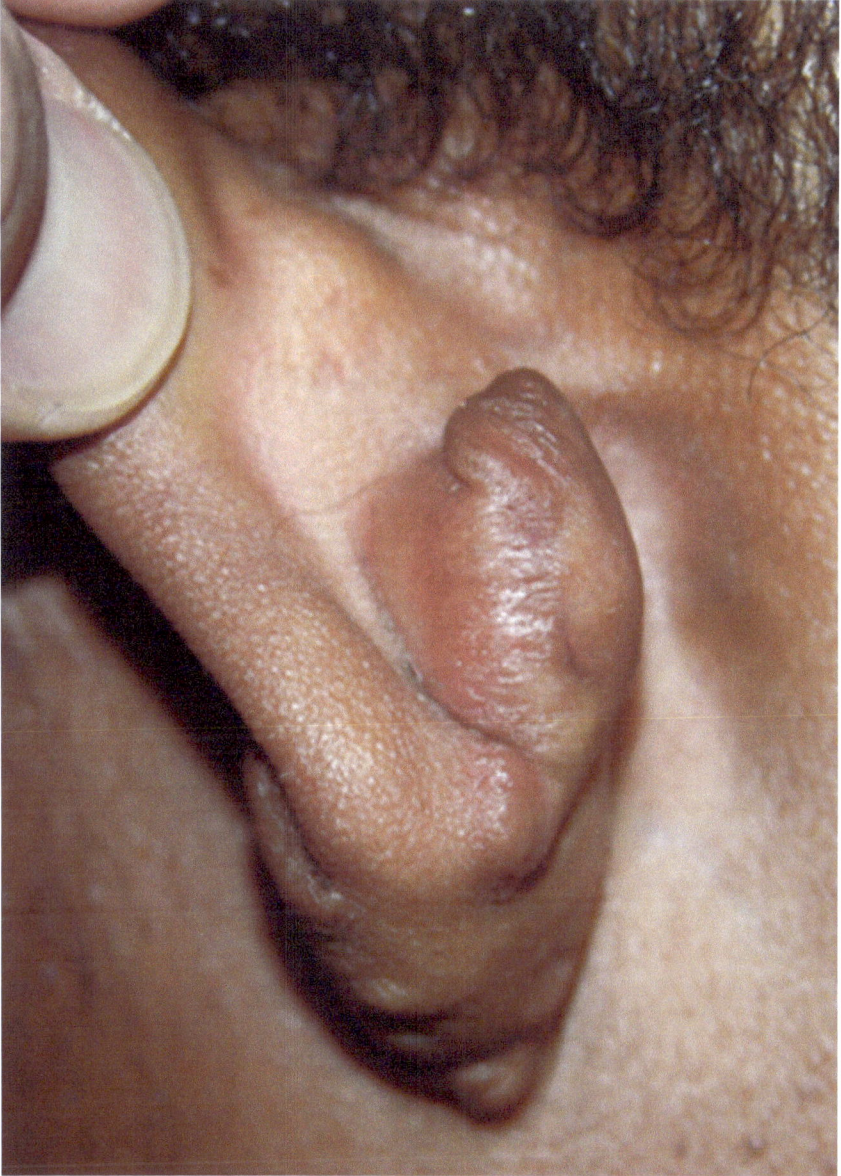

Fig. 57: Recurrence of keloid after multiple surgeries. Notice the keloid regrowth on both surfaces of the earlobe. Posterior view of the patient depicted in *Fig. 56.*

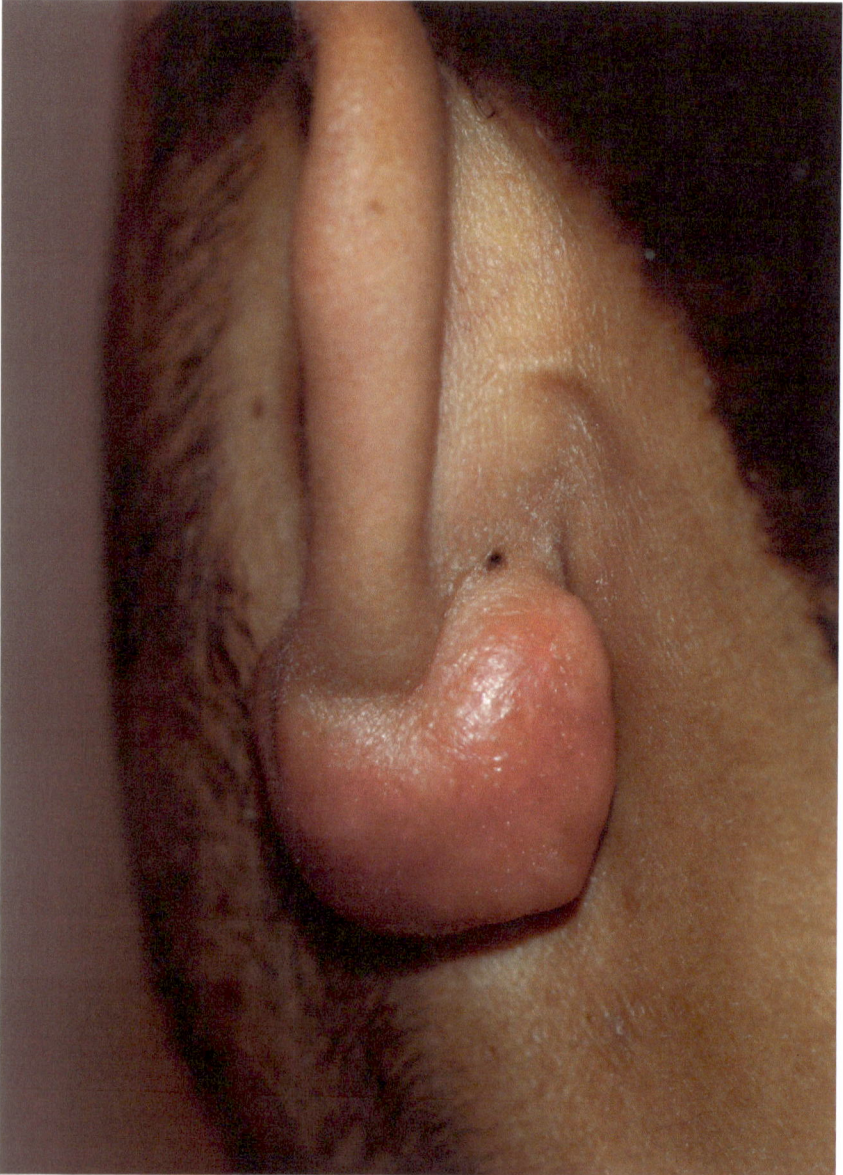

Fig. 58: Tumoral recurrence of keloid after total removal of the left earlobe.

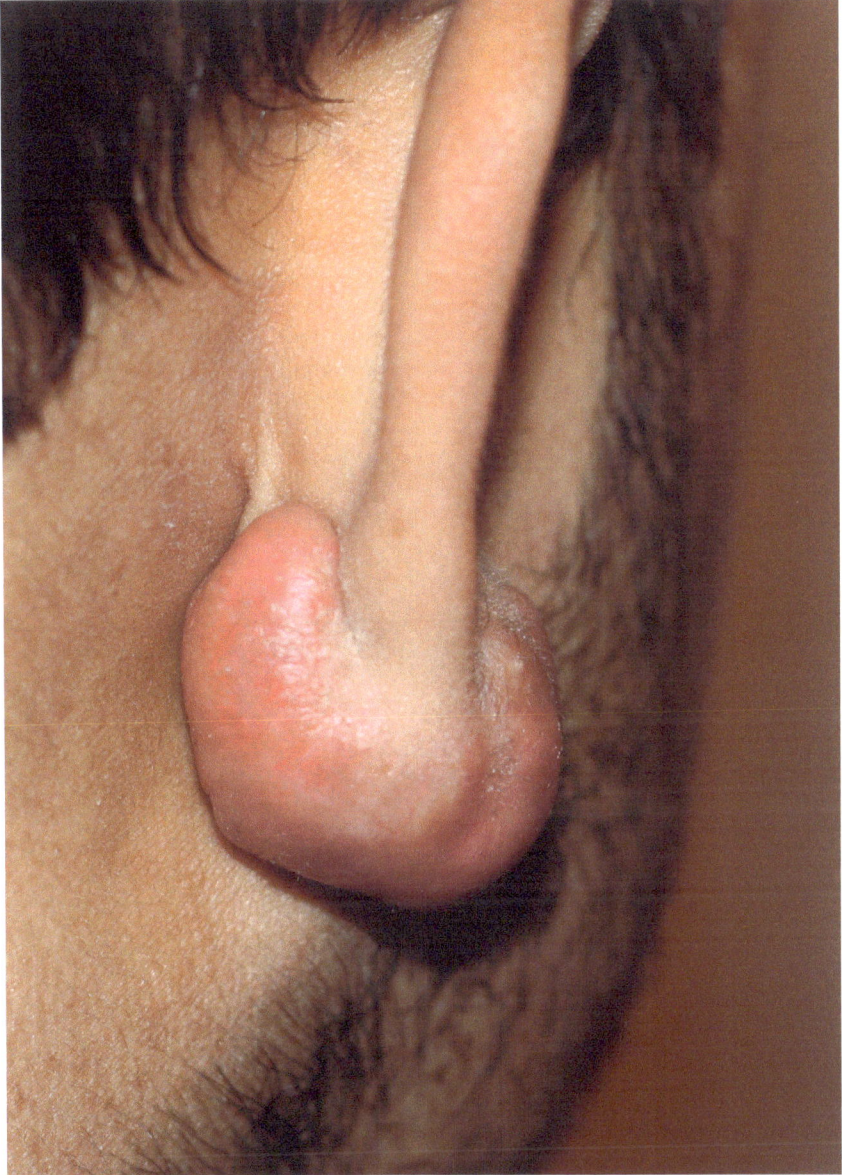

Fig. 59: Near symmetrical tumoral recurrence of keloid after total removal of the right earlobe in the same patient depicted in *Fig. 58.*

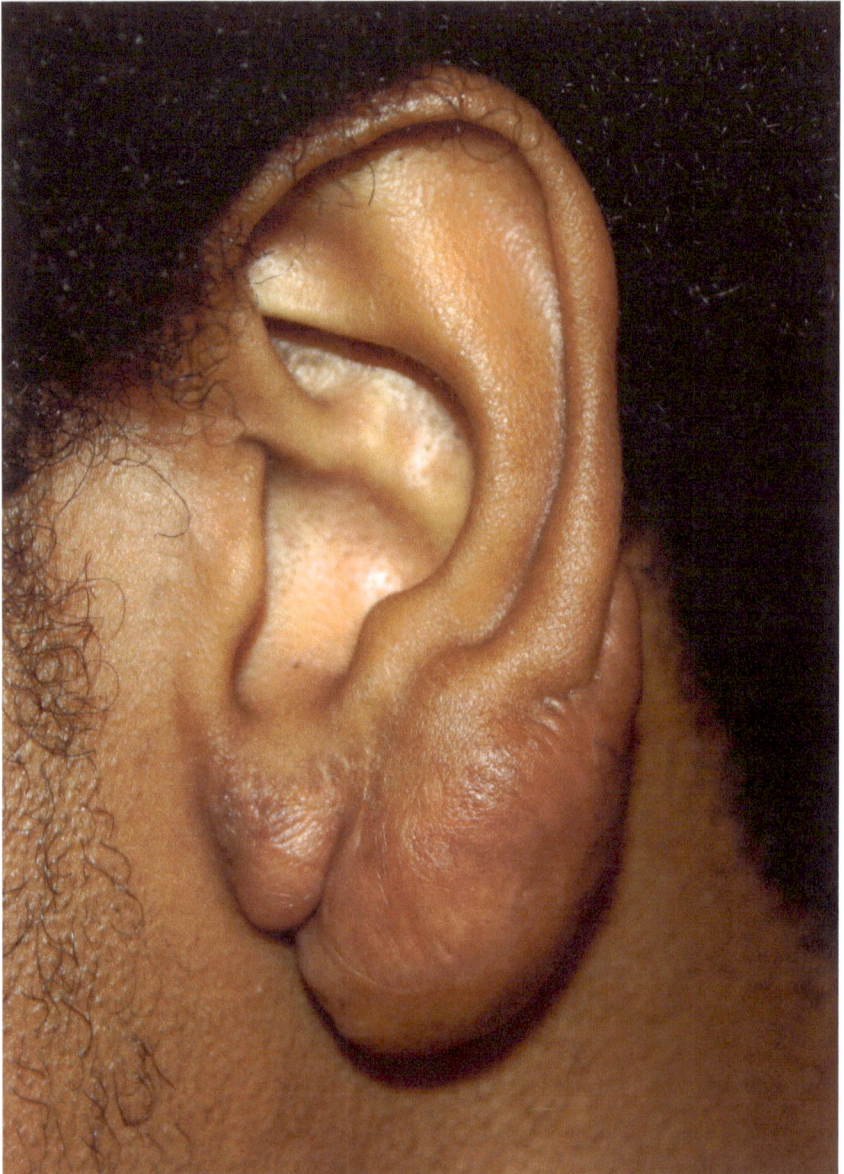

Fig. 60: Tumoral recurrence of keloid after total removal of the left earlobe.

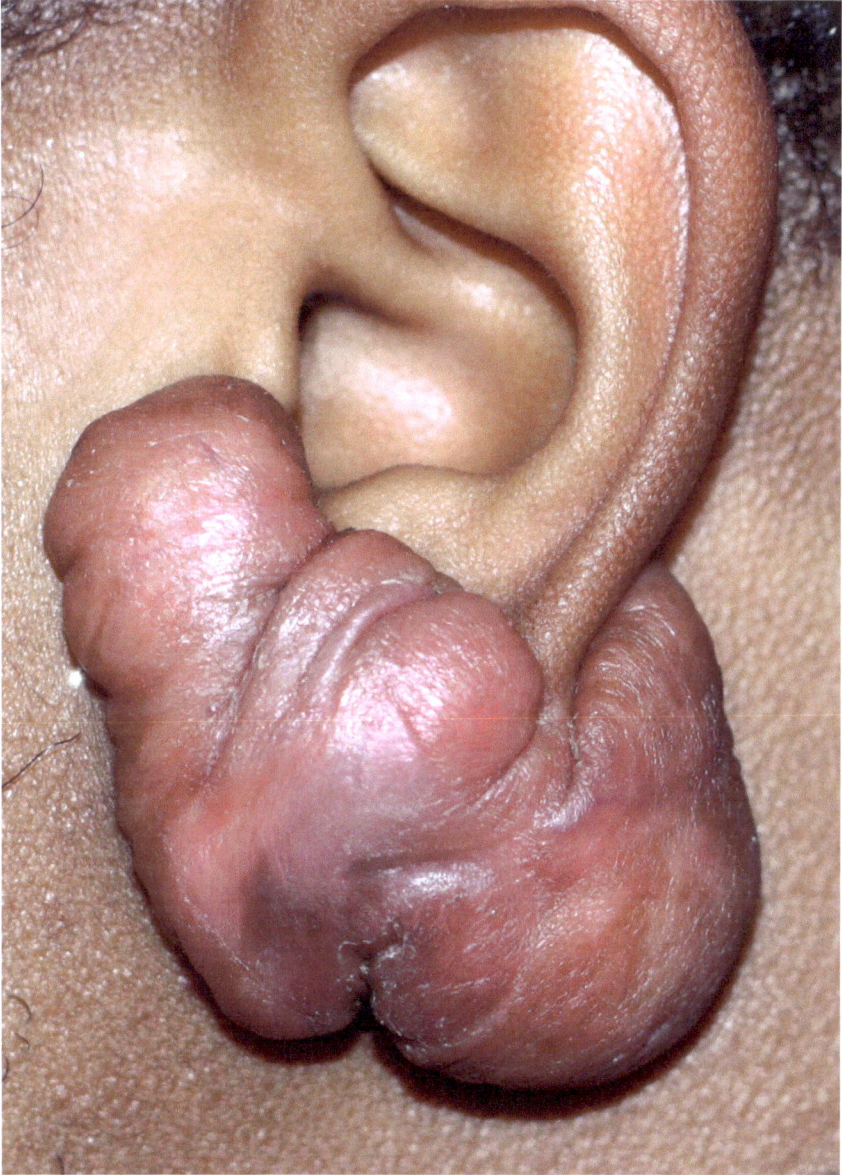

Fig. 61: Very large tumoral recurrence of keloid after surgical removal of the left earlobe. Notice the multi-directional aggressive growth pattern of secondary keloid, a growth pattern that is only seen in secondary keloids.

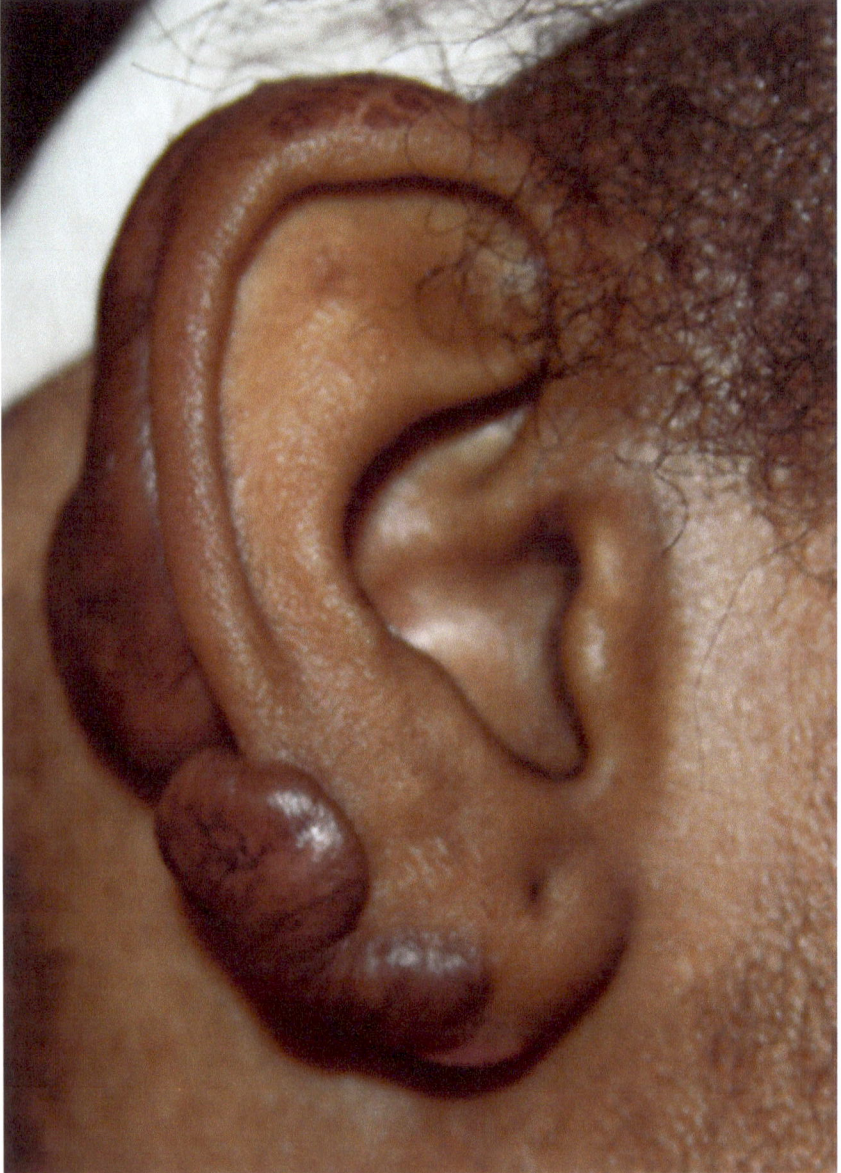

Fig. 62: Very advanced local recurrence of ear keloid involving much of the ear. Notice lack of keloid formation in the anterior surface of the earlobe at the site of ear piercing.

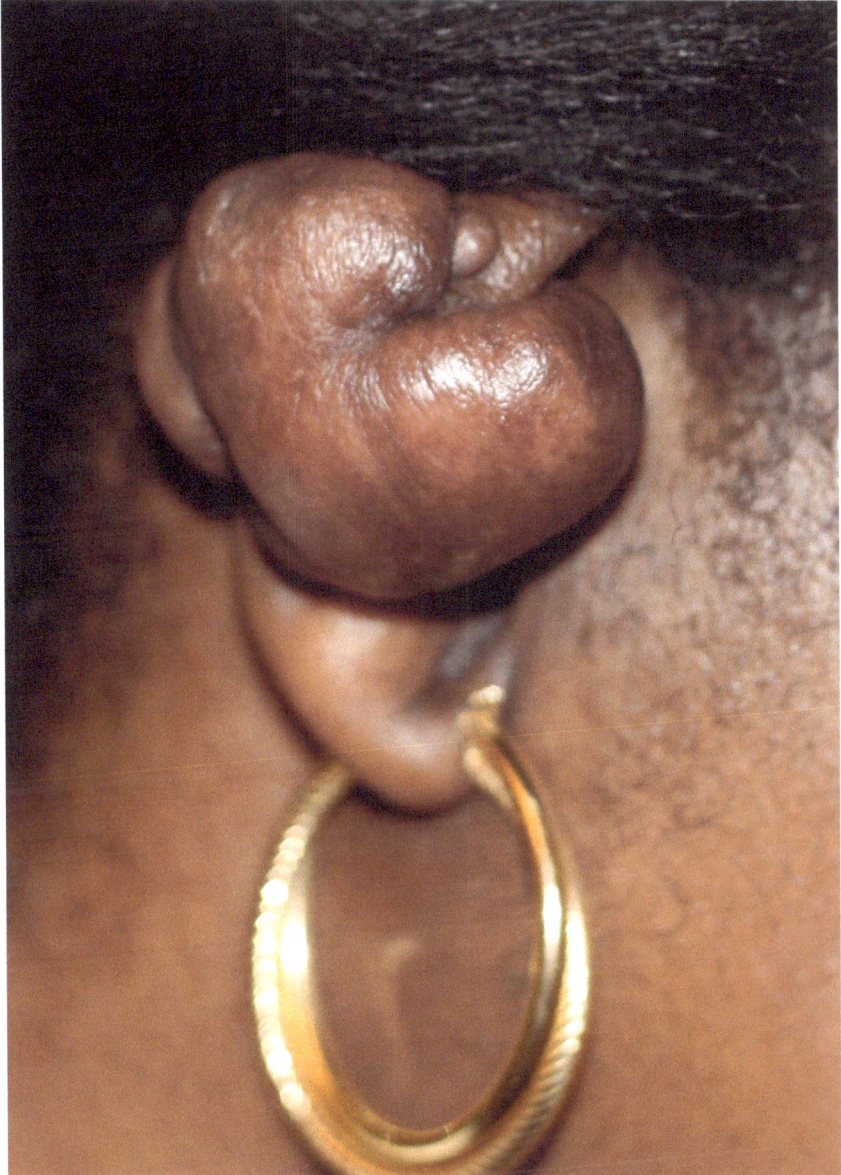

Fig. 63: Disfiguring recurrence of ear keloid after surgery in a twenty-five year-old female. The weight of the secondary keloid has caused the helix of her ear to fold and be pulled down to cover her ear canal, interfering with her hearing ability.

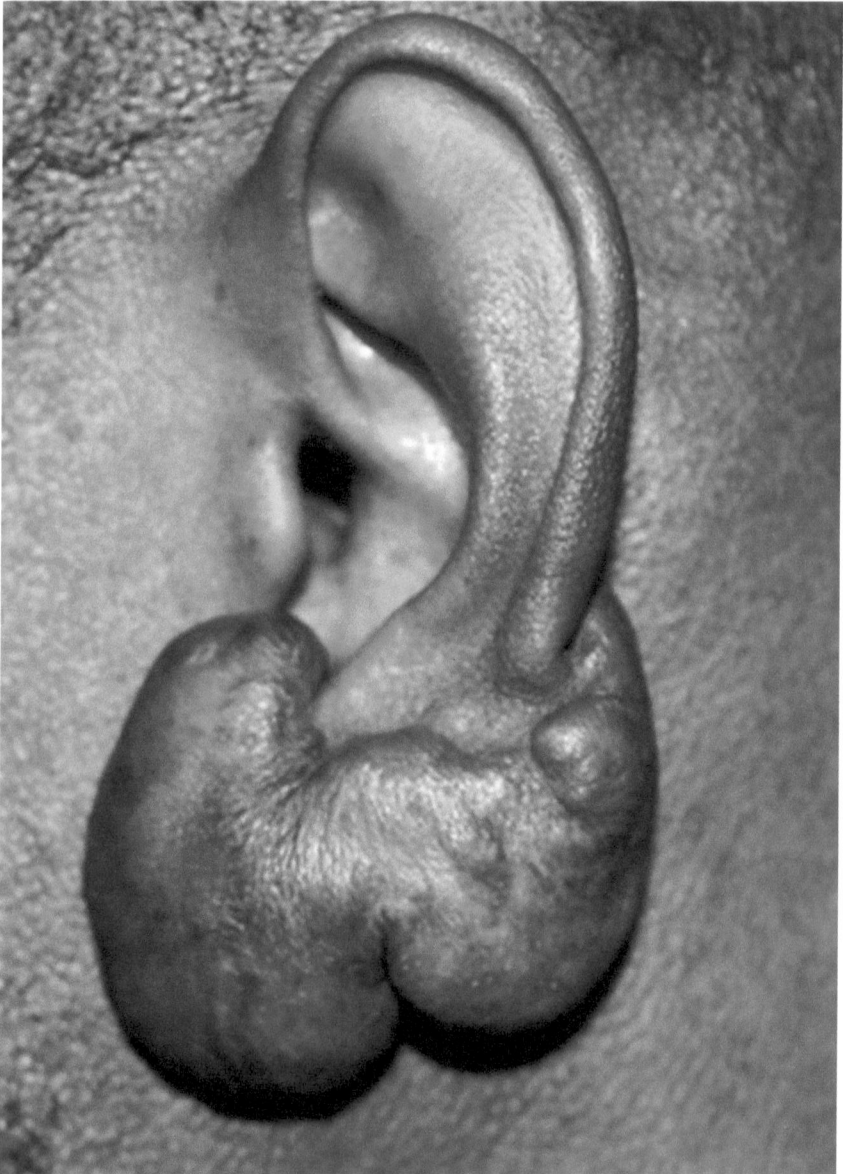

Fig. 64: Disfiguring recurrence of ear keloid after surgery. Note the clear absence of the earlobe, which is due to prior surgical resection to treat the primary keloid. Also note the expansion of the keloid towards the ear canal, as well as forward expansion away from the ear.

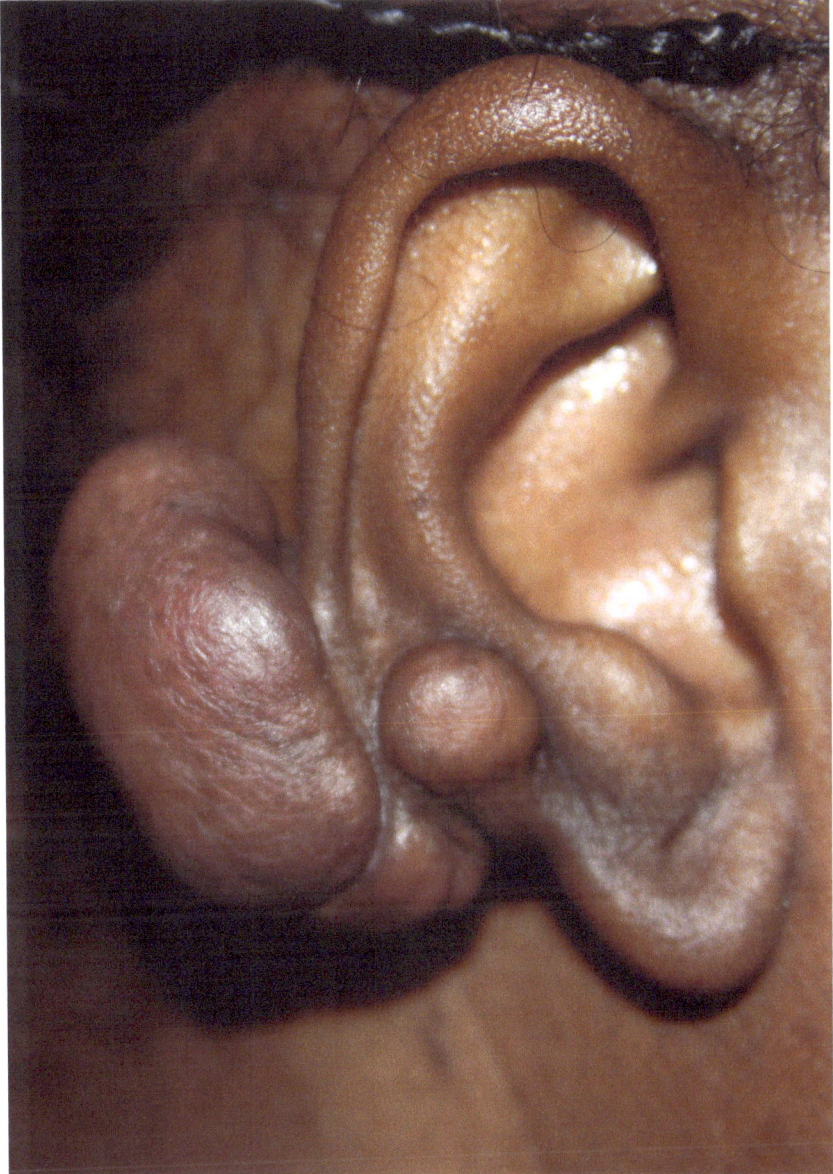

Fig. 65: Disfiguring recurrence of ear keloid after surgery. Note the upward growth of the larger keloid and a separate keloid nodule on the anterior surface of the ear.

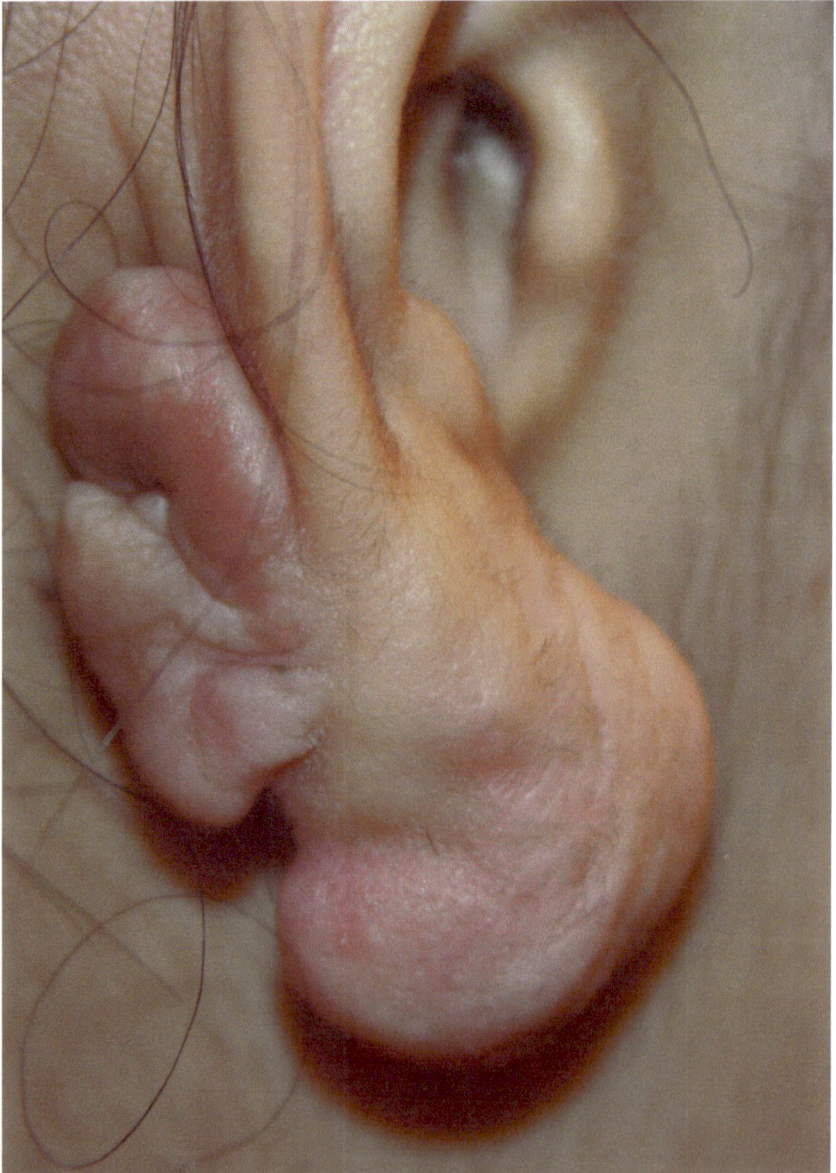

Fig. 66: Disfiguring recurrence of ear keloid after multiple surgical attempts. Lack of control of keloids with repeated surgery results in patient frustration and withdrawal from medical care. Most patients depicted here have given up on treatment and have decided to live with the nightmare imposed on them by disfiguring recurrences after surgery.

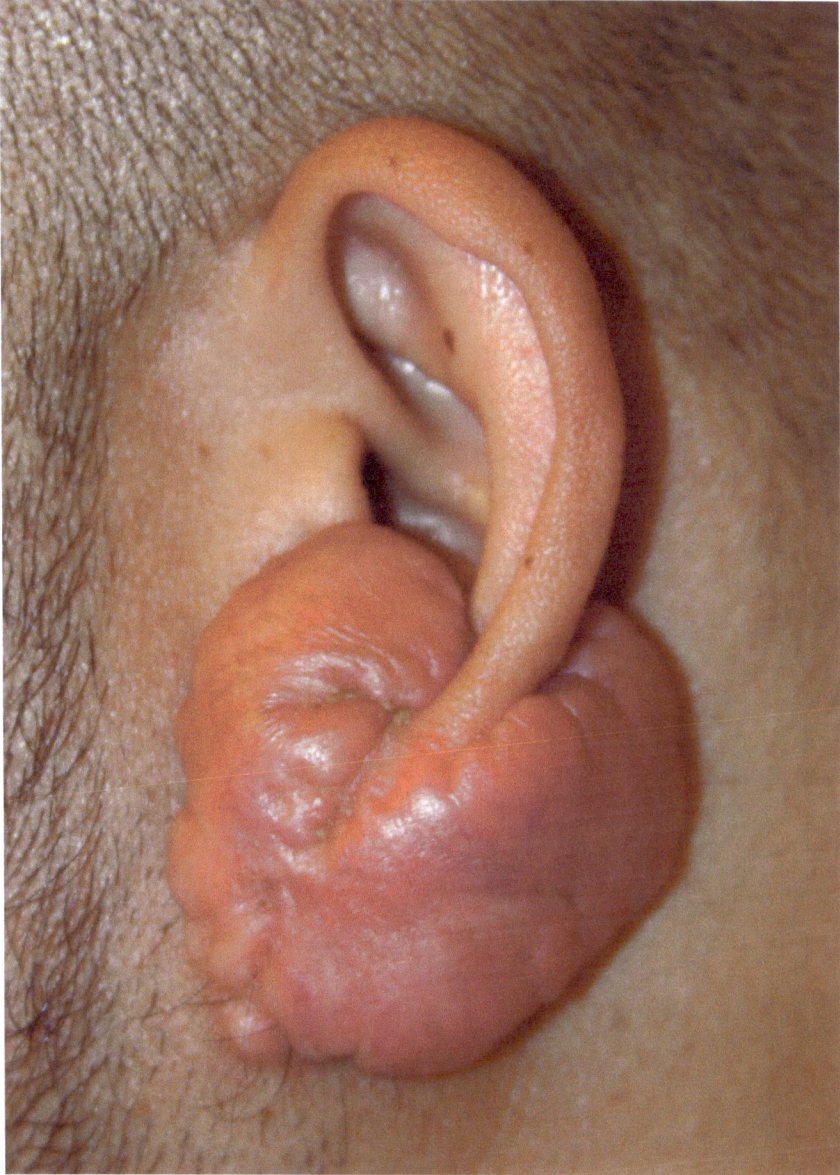

Fig. 67: Disfiguring recurrence of ear keloid after surgery. Note the invasive nature of the keloid and its aggressive expansion and engulfing of the ear; a feature unique to secondary keloids that is never seen in primary keloids.

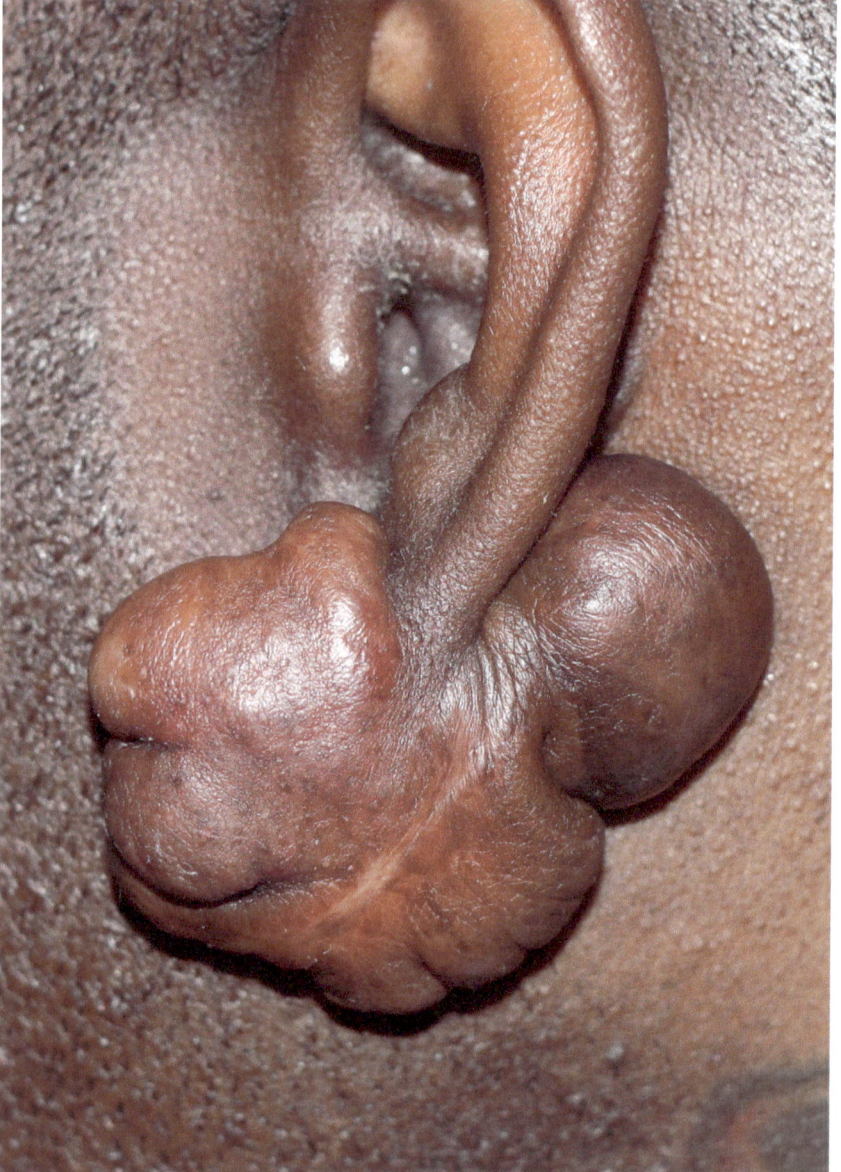

Fig. 68: A very disfiguring recurrent earlobe keloid after a failed surgery. Note the tumoral expansion and engulfing of the earlobe; a feature unique to secondary keloids.

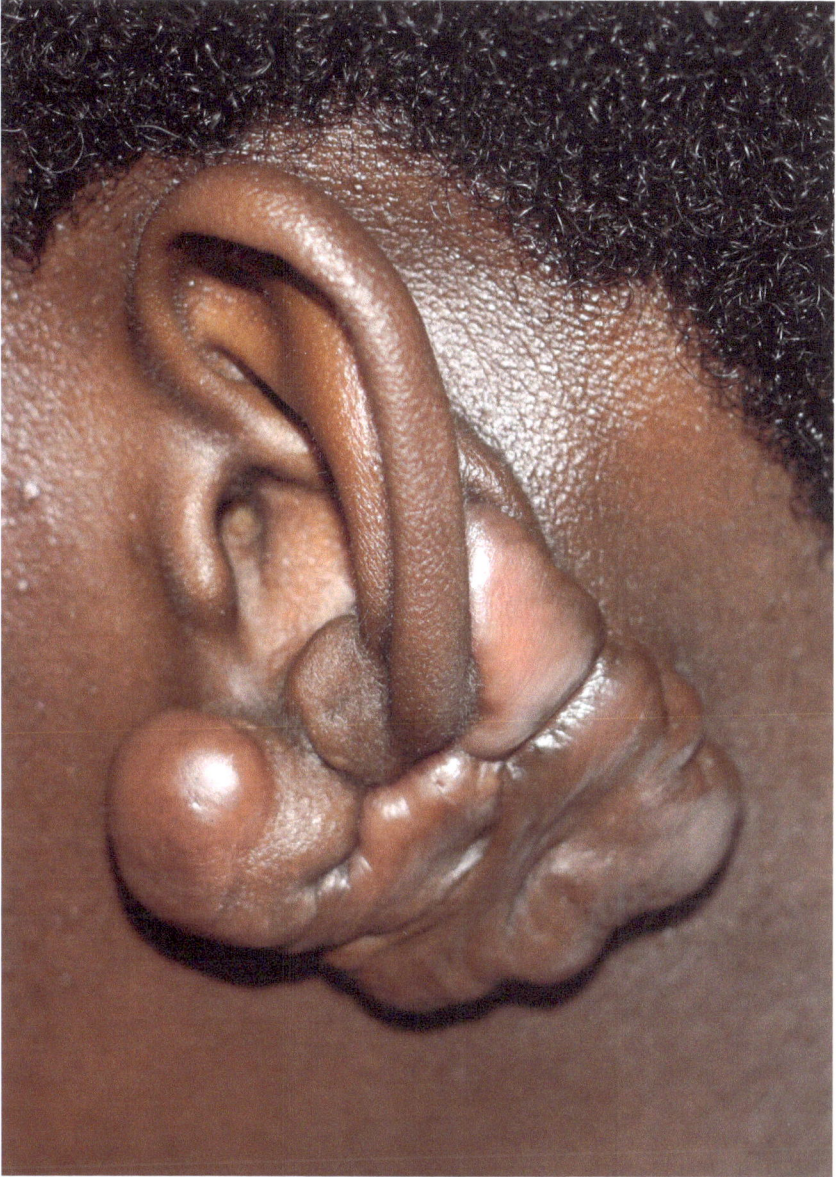

Fig. 69: Disfiguring recurrence of ear keloid after multiple surgeries.

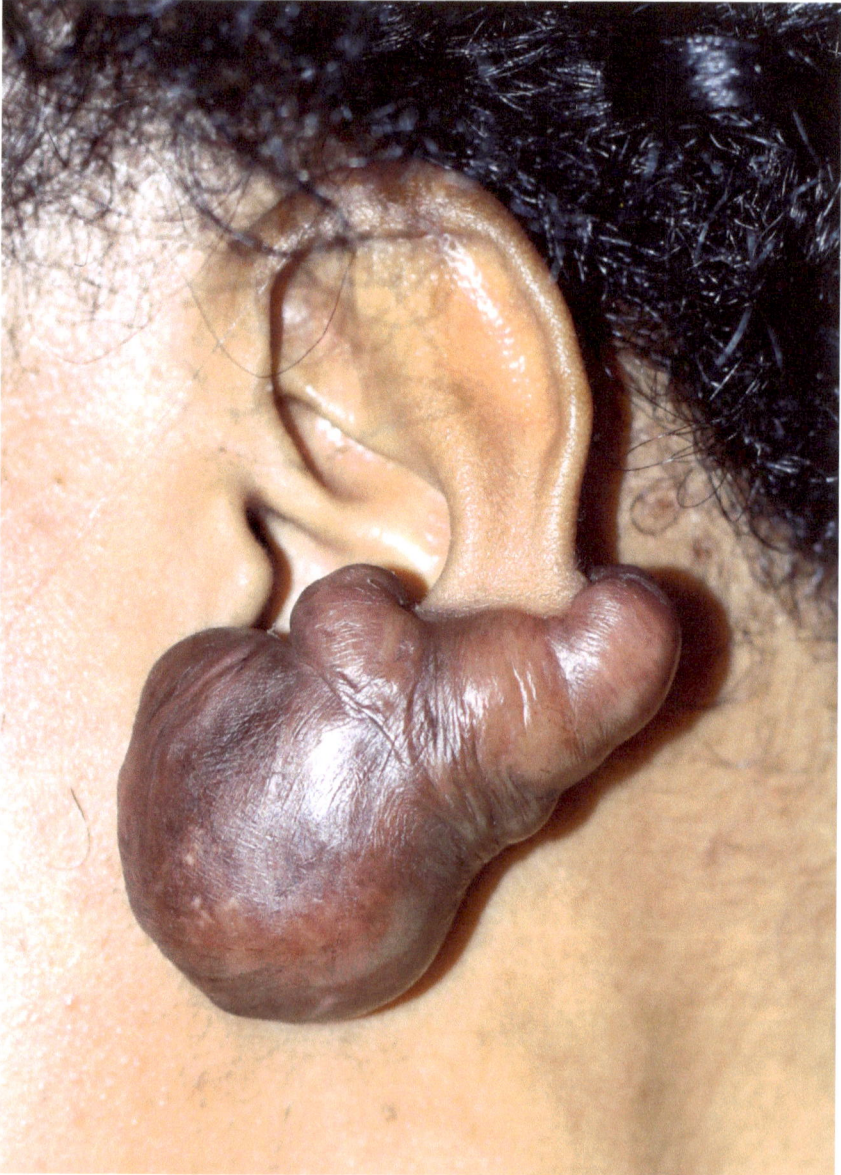

Fig. 70: Disfiguring and tumoral recurrence of ear keloid after multiple surgeries to remove an earlobe keloid. Note the expansion of the keloid towards the ear canal.

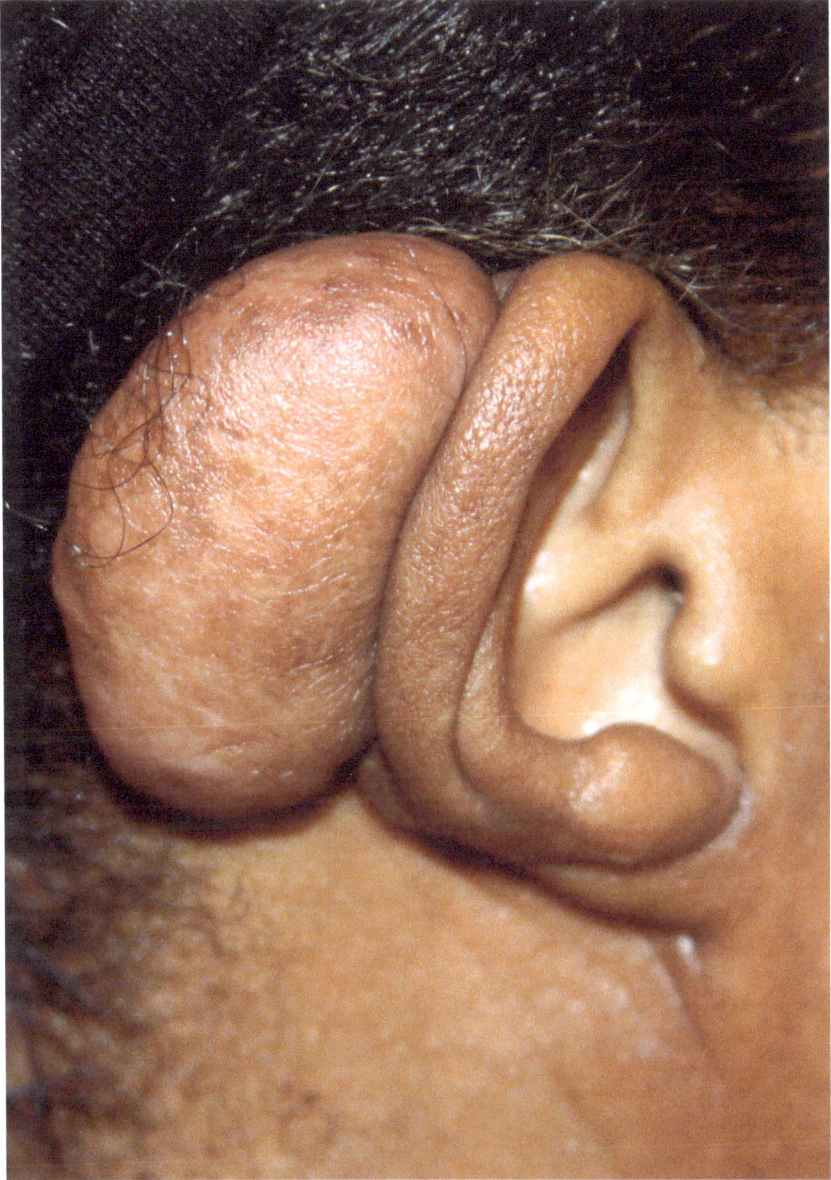

Fig. 71: Large tumoral recurrence of ear keloid in posterior surface of the ear. Note the absence of the earlobe from a prior surgery.

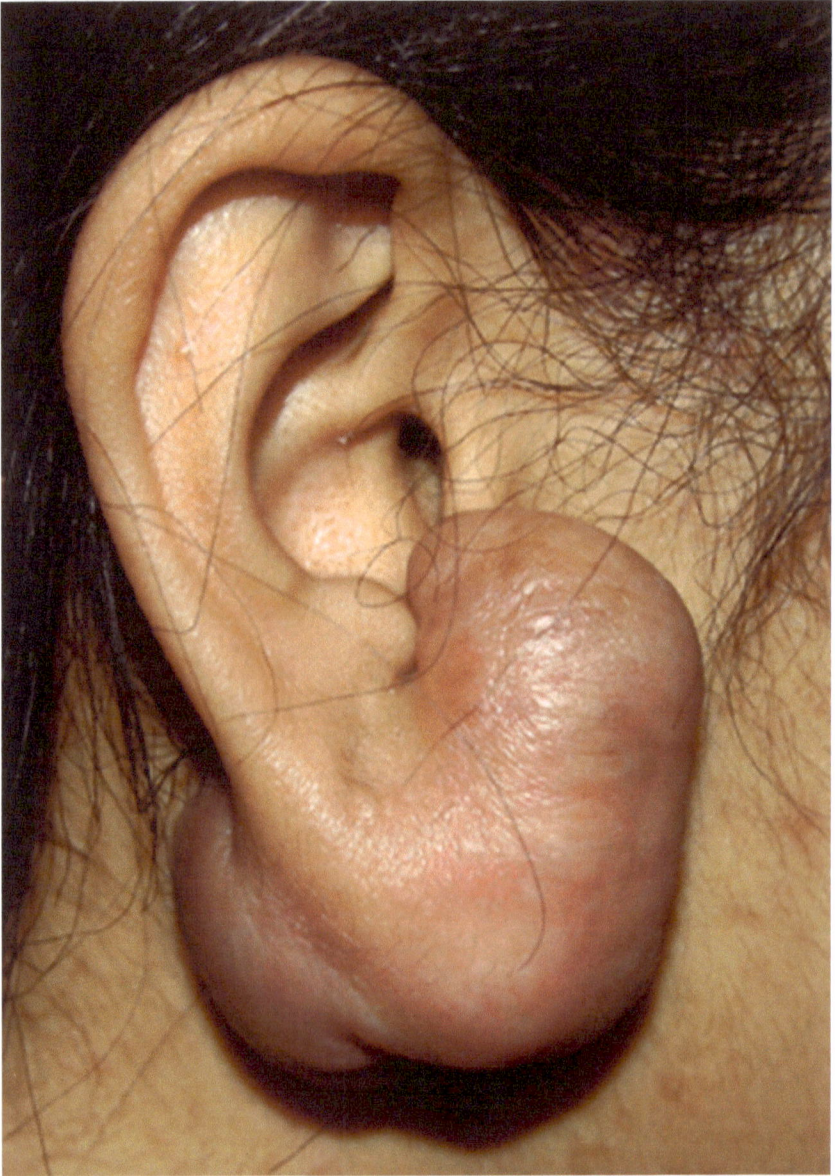

Fig. 72: Disfiguring recurrence of ear keloid after multiple surgeries. Note the expansion of the keloid process towards the ear canal.

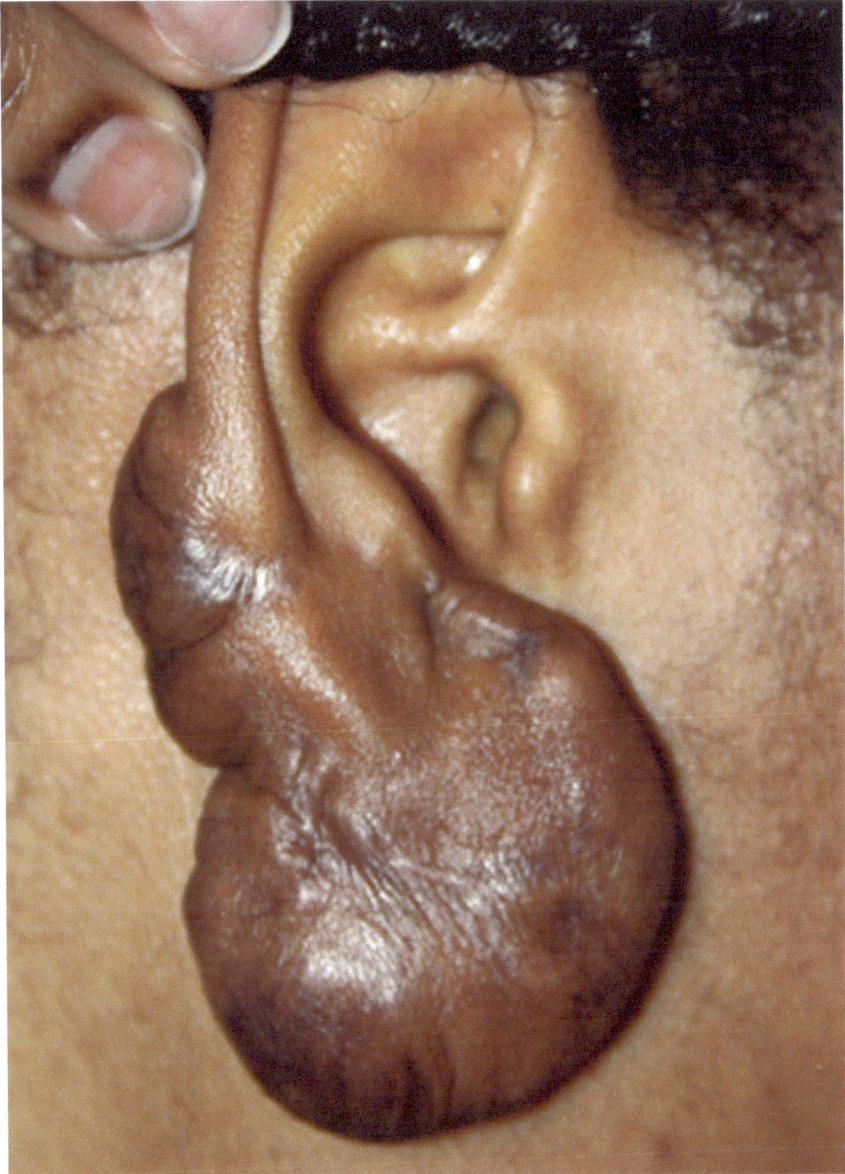

Fig. 73: Disfiguring recurrence of ear keloid after multiple surgeries. Note total absence of earlobe, growth and local expansion of the keloid.

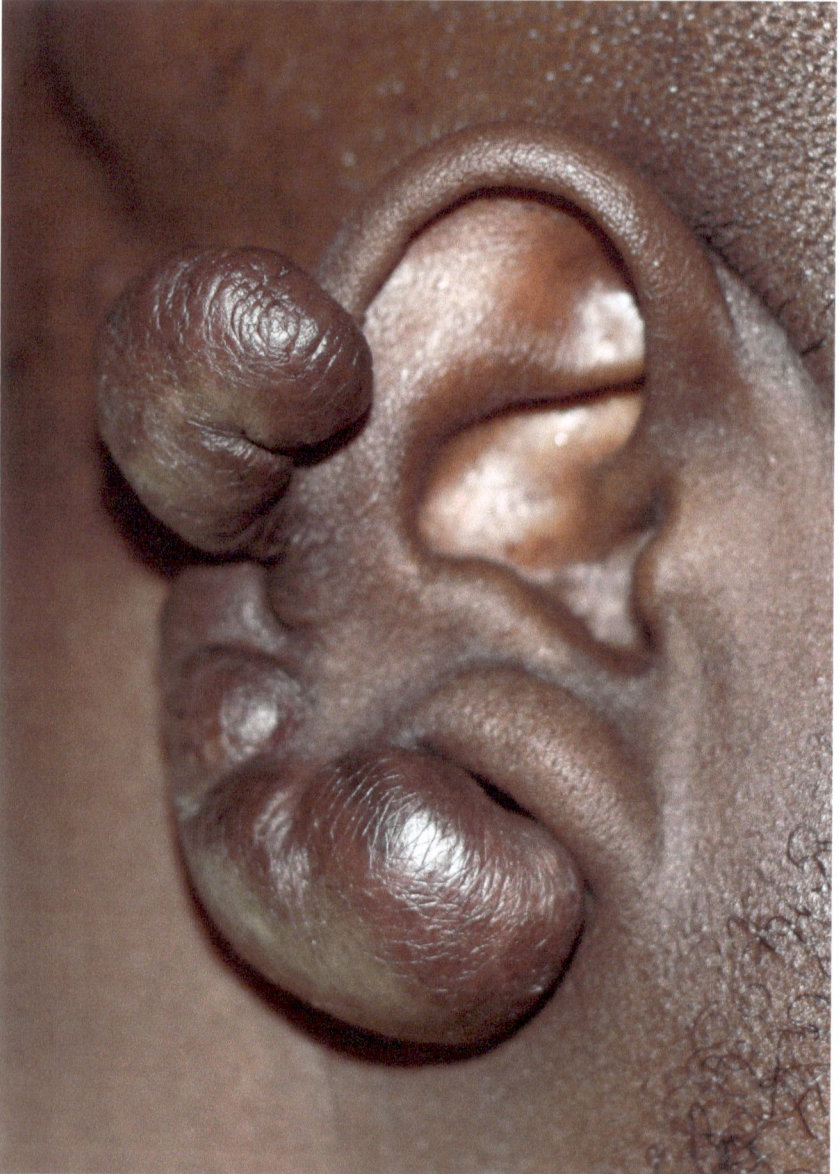

Fig. 74: Disfiguring tumoral recurrence of ear keloids after multiple surgeries.

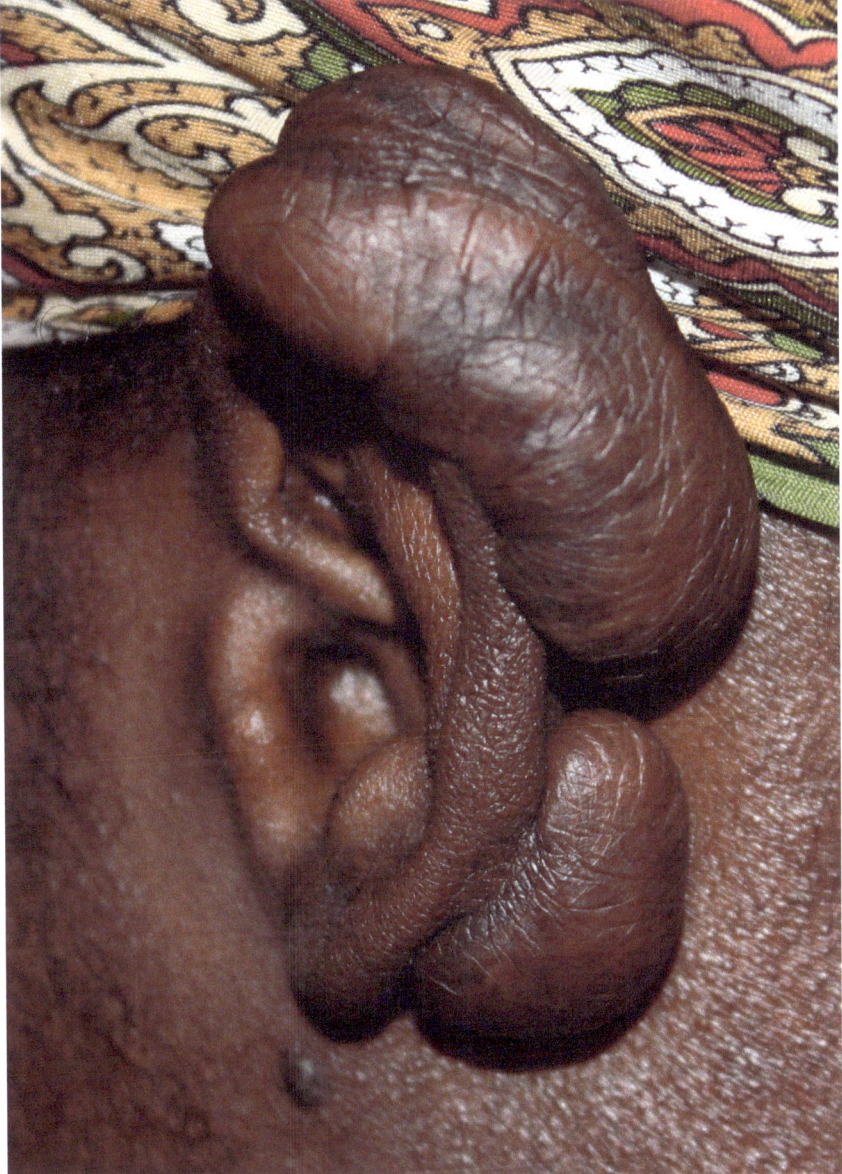

Fig. 75: Disfiguring tumoral recurrence of ear keloids after multiple surgeries.

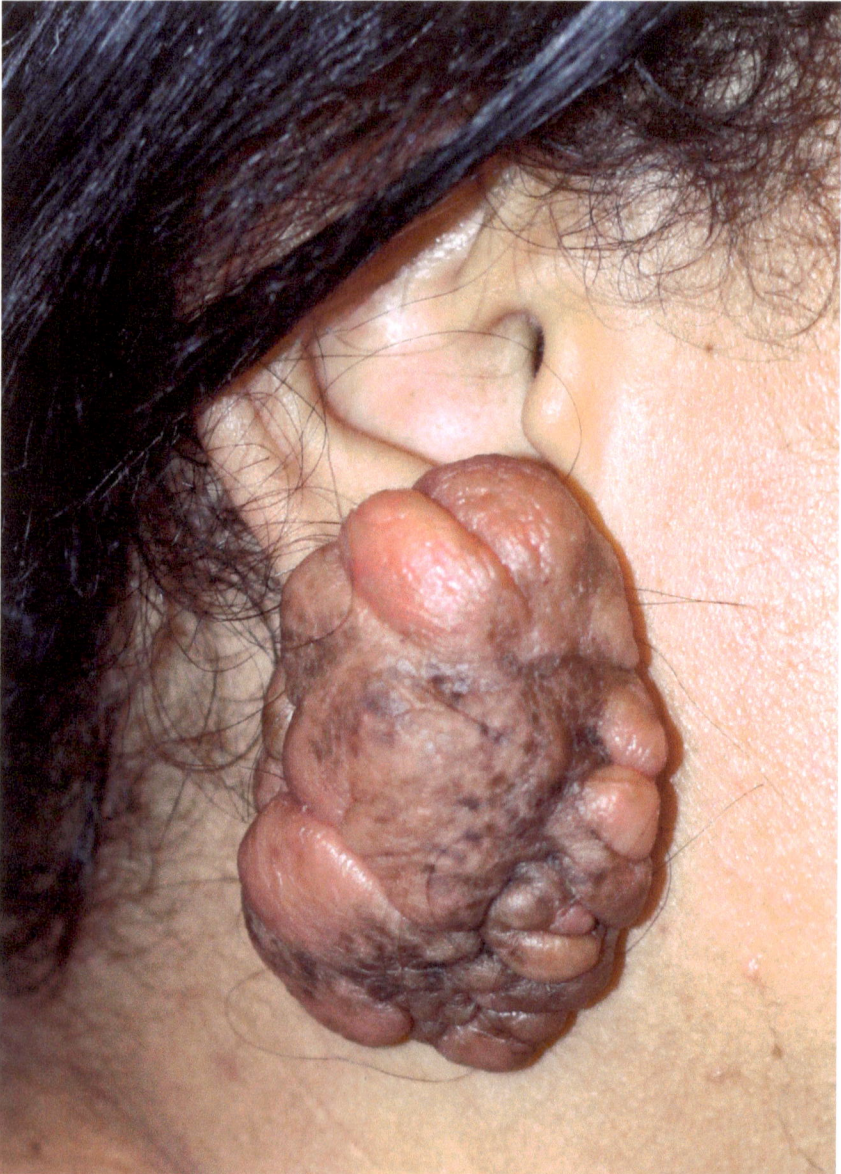

Fig. 76: Disfiguring tumoral recurrence of ear keloids after multiple surgeries. This patient rejected repeat surgery and chose to simply cover her ear with her luckily thick hair.

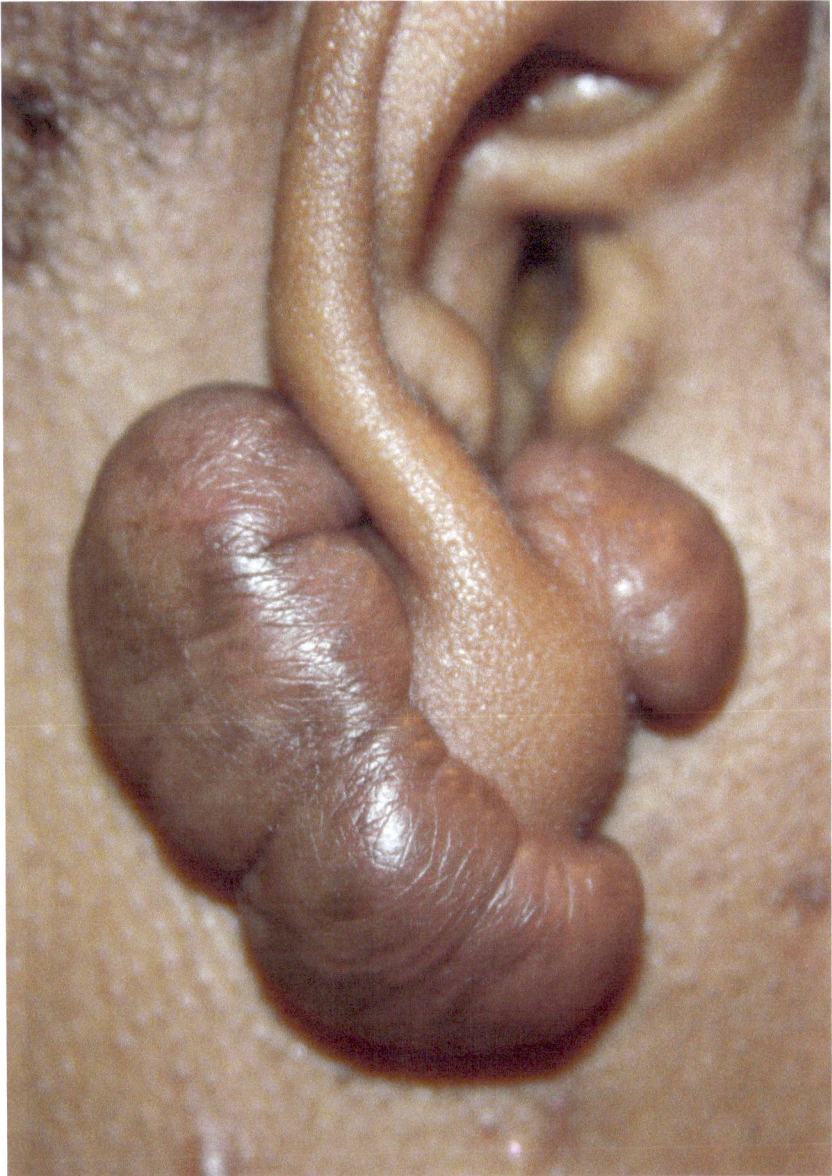

Fig. 77: Disfiguring tumoral recurrence of ear keloids after multiple surgeries.

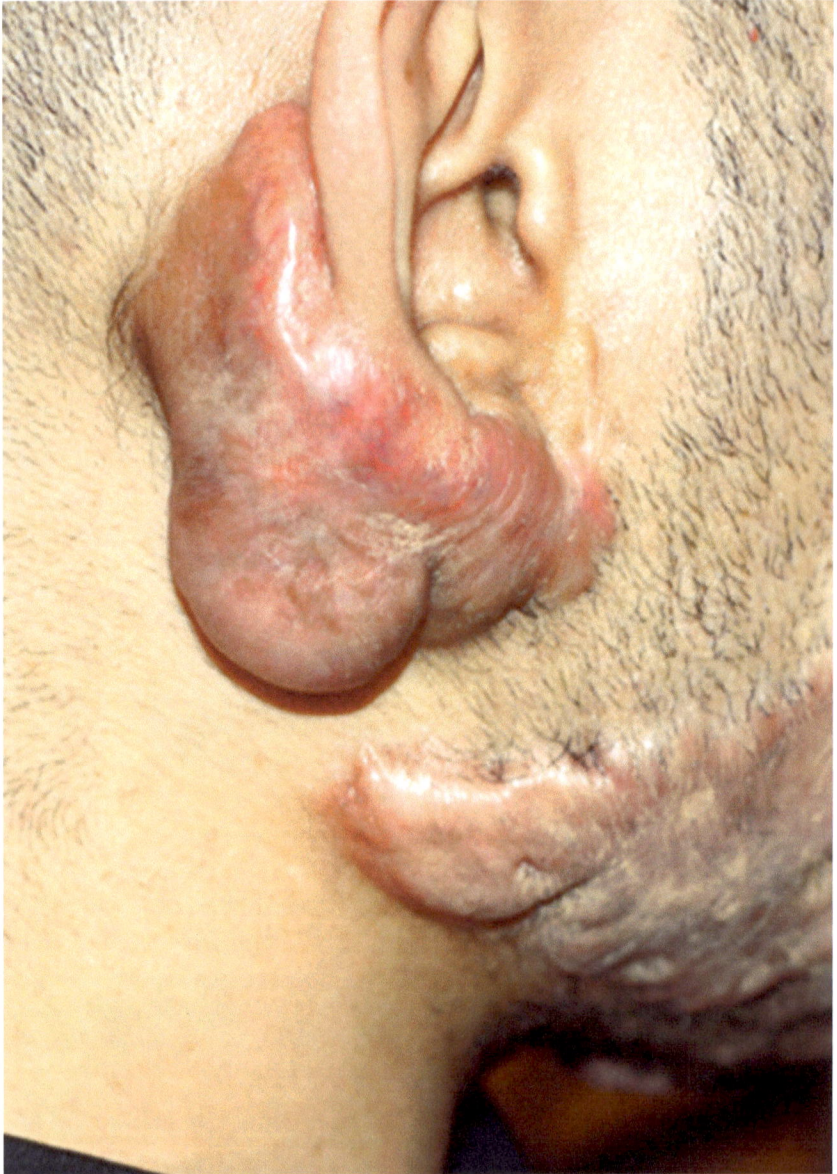

Fig. 78: Disfiguring tumoral recurrence of ear keloids after multiple surgeries. Note the presence of facial keloids. Despite all recurrences, this patient was once again offered another round of surgery by a surgeon.

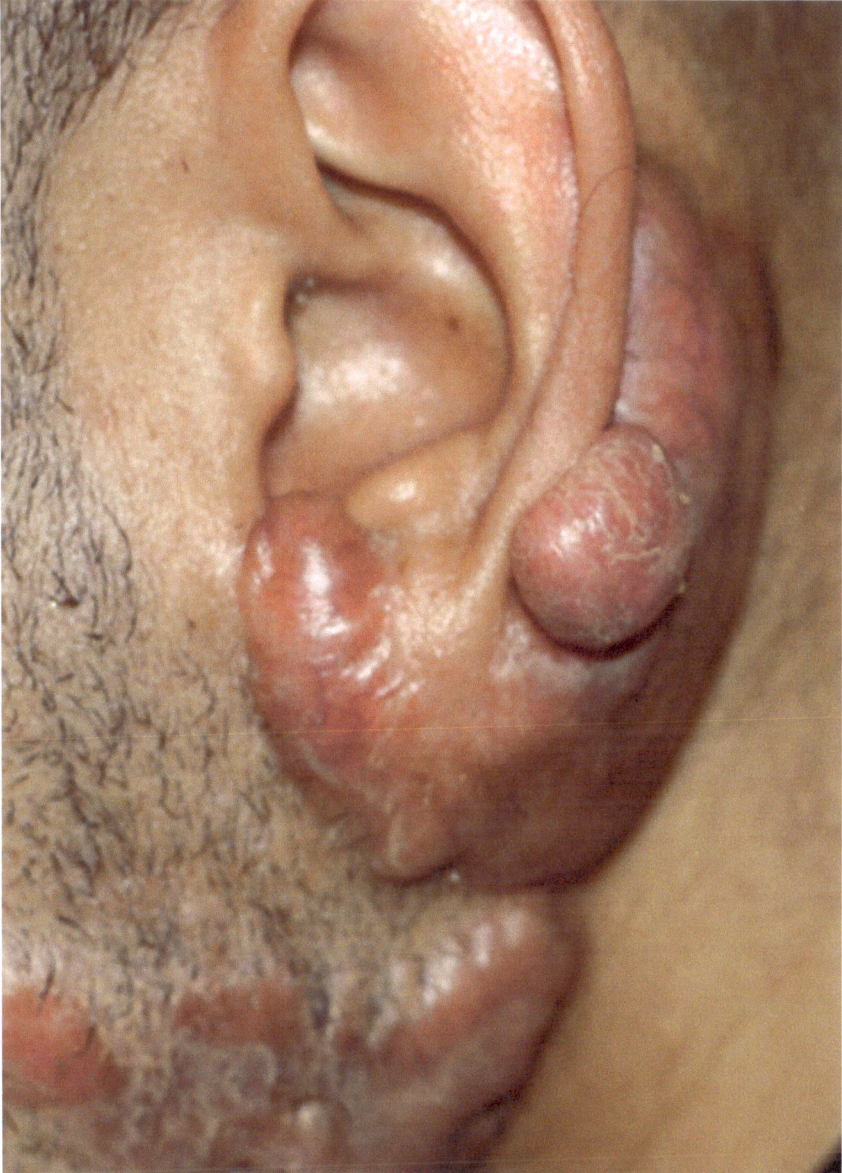

Fig. 79: Disfiguring tumoral recurrence of left ear keloids after multiple surgeries in the same patient as depicted in *Fig. 78*. This type of recurrence is commonly seen in patients who have keloids on other parts of their skin.

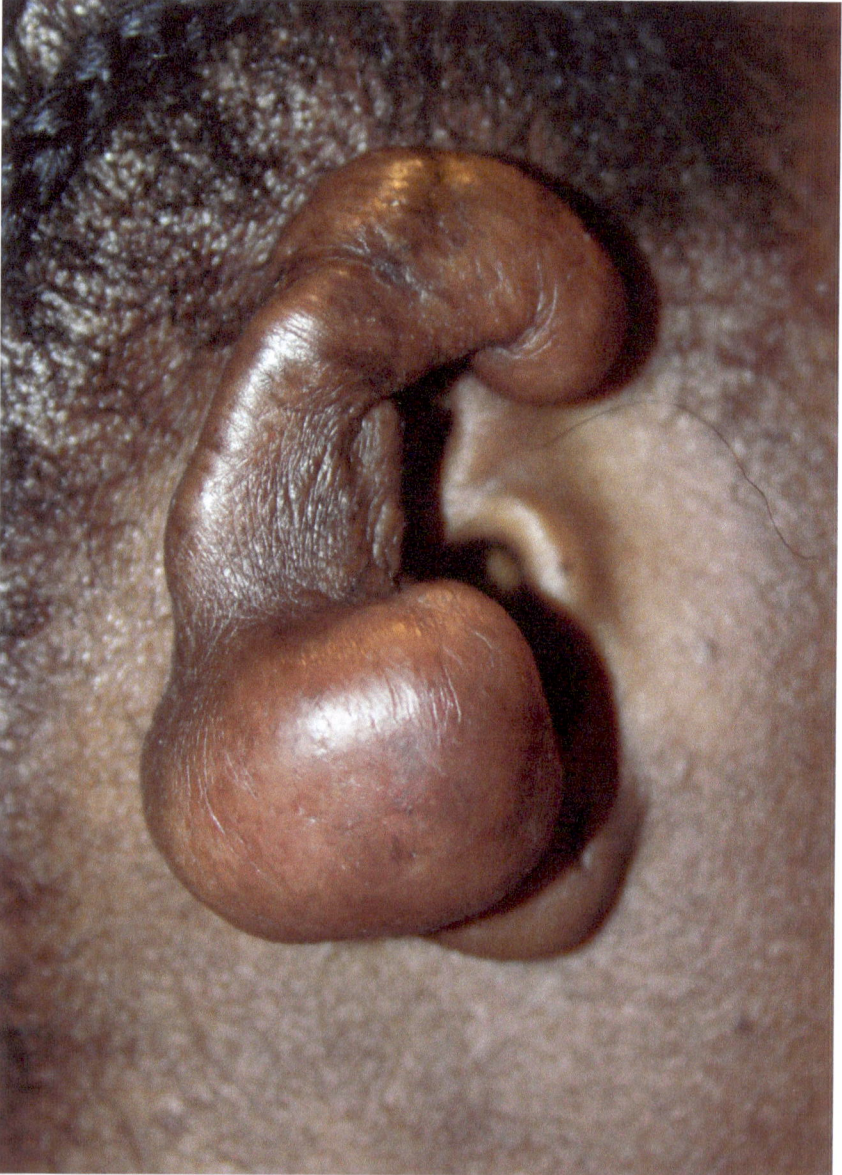

Fig. 80: Disfiguring tumoral recurrence of ear keloids after multiple surgeries. Note the near-total involvement of the right ear with the keloid process.

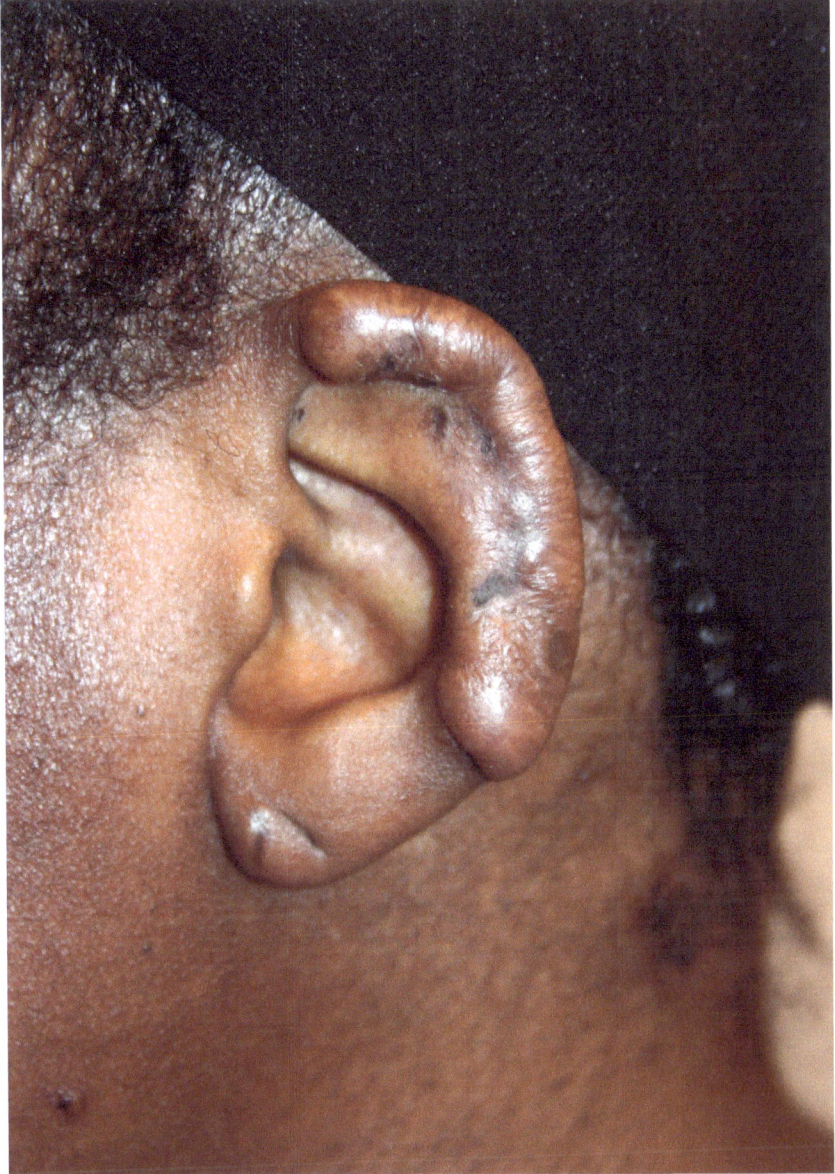

Fig. 81: Disfiguring tumoral recurrence of ear keloids after multiple surgeries. Note the near total-destruction of the left helix of the ear with the keloid process.

5 MASSIVE EAR KELOIDS

MASSIVE EAR KELOIDS often form after multiple surgical attempts to remove a secondary keloid. It is the constant, indiscriminate damage and injury to the ear tissue by repeated surgeries that results in a terrible recurrence. Unfortunately, there are still some patients who are subjected to repeated surgery to remove secondary keloids.

Massive ear keloids are almost exclusively seen in African Americans and in those with dark skin color. The author has not seen massive keloids among Whites or Caucasians.

The constant worsening of the keloids frustrates the patients, who unfortunately find nowhere to go, other than from one surgeon to the next, who will inevitably recommend more surgeries.

Most patients with large or massive keloids realize, at some point, that repeated surgeries will only worsen their condition and decide to live with their keloids, and allow them to grow. The rate of growth of these keloids is much faster than any primary keloid.

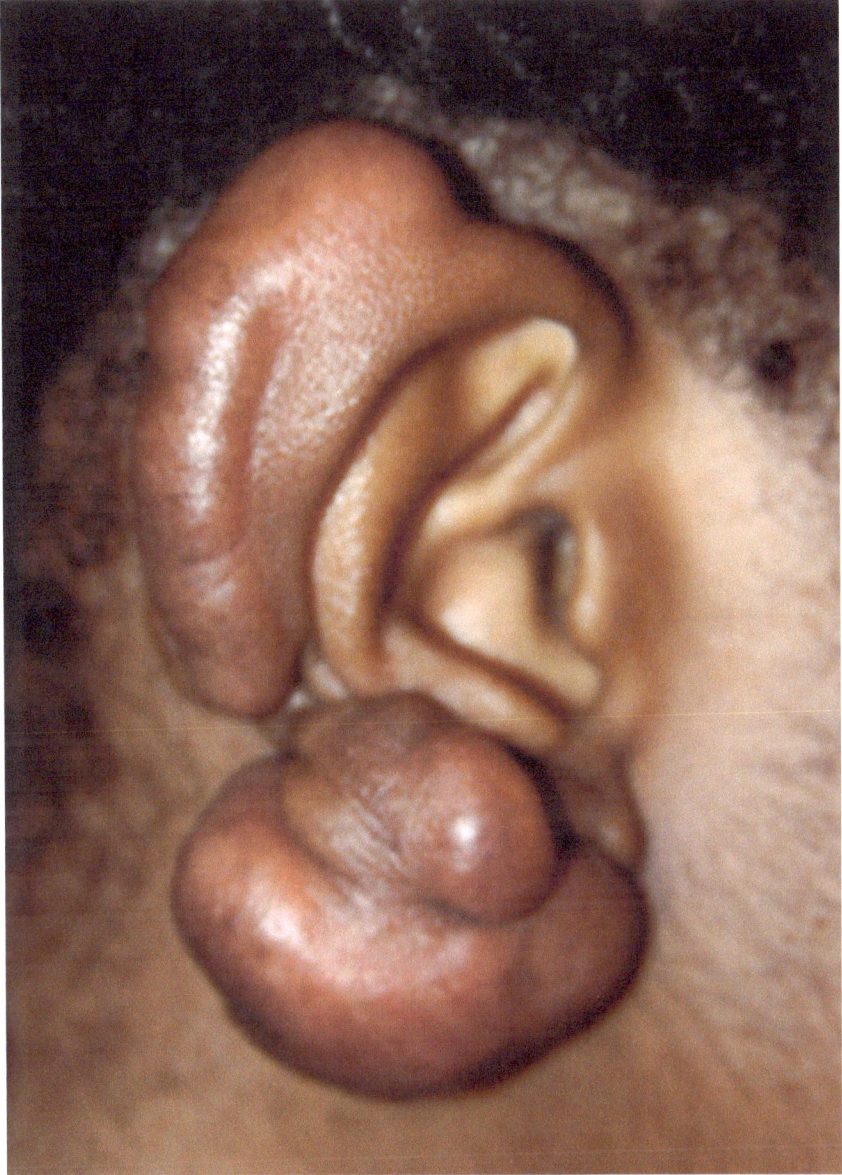

Fig. 82: Massive ear keloids

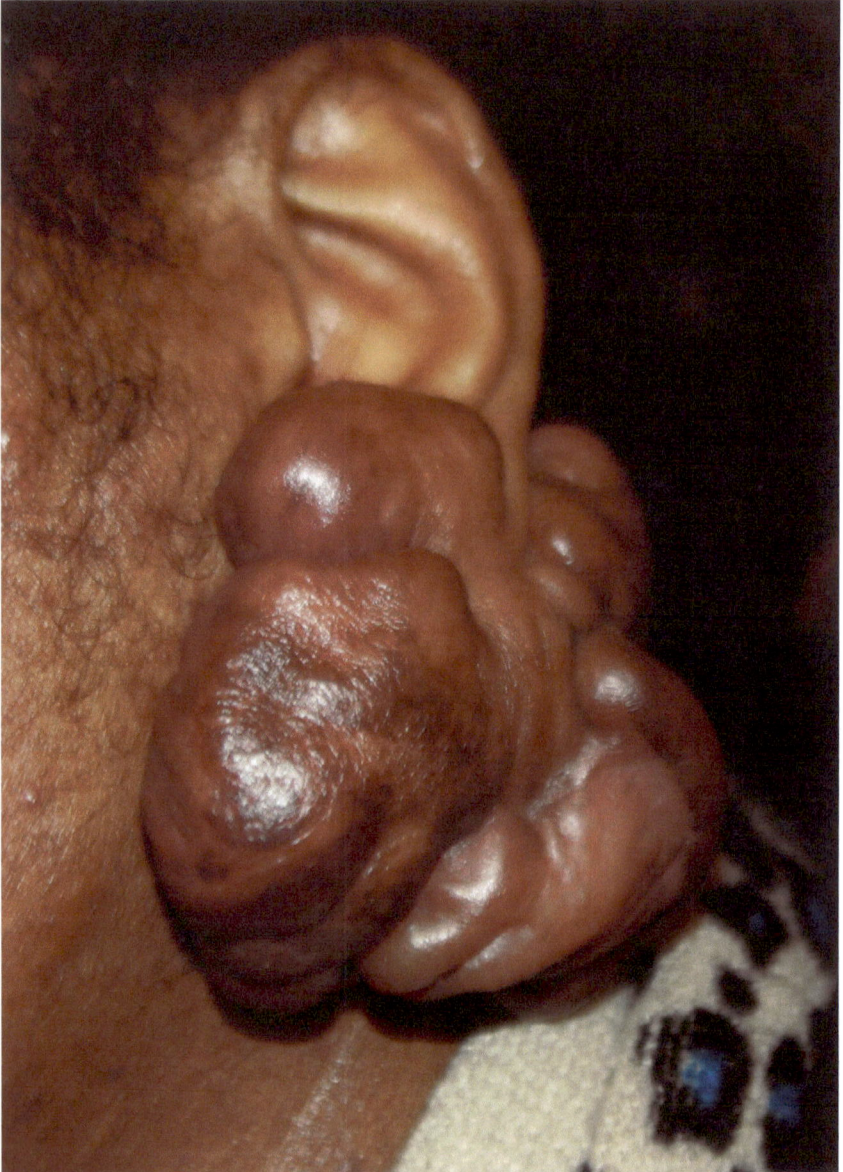

Fig. 83: Massive ear keloids in a college student. Patients like this young woman have very low self-esteem, hardly have any friends, and are constantly subjected to queries and ridicule from others. They often cover their hair, and their ears, with either a wig or a hat.

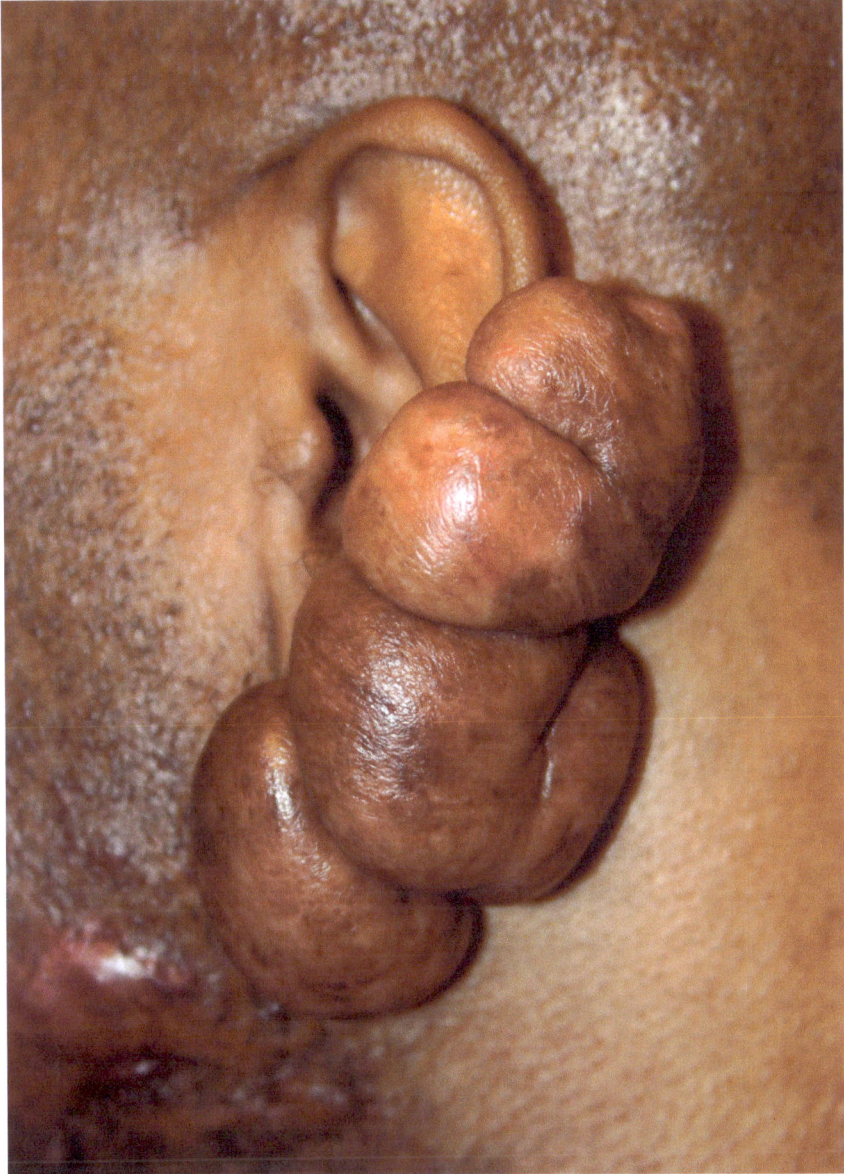

Fig. 84: Massive ear keloids in a young male. Patients like this young man encounter prejudice in the work place, have a hard time succeeding in job interviews and often wear hoodies to hide their keloid(s).

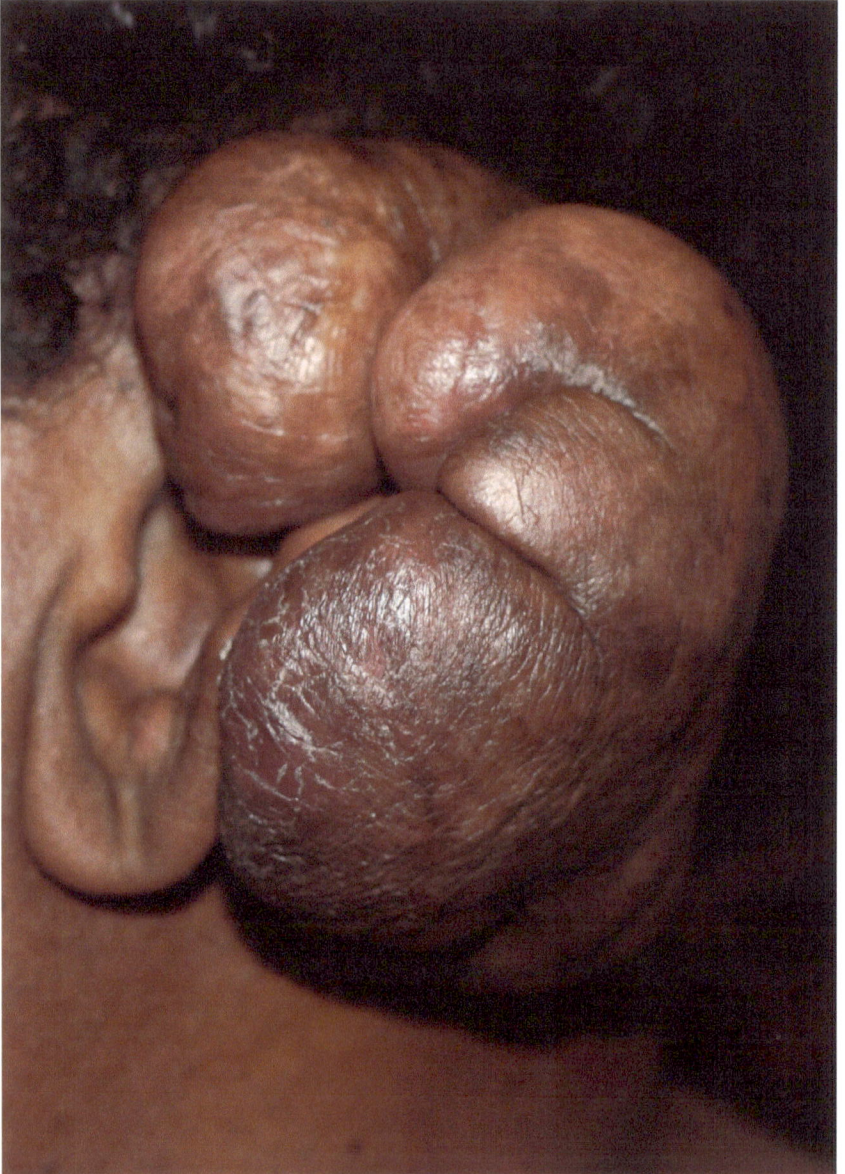

Fig. 85: Massive ear keloids in a young male.

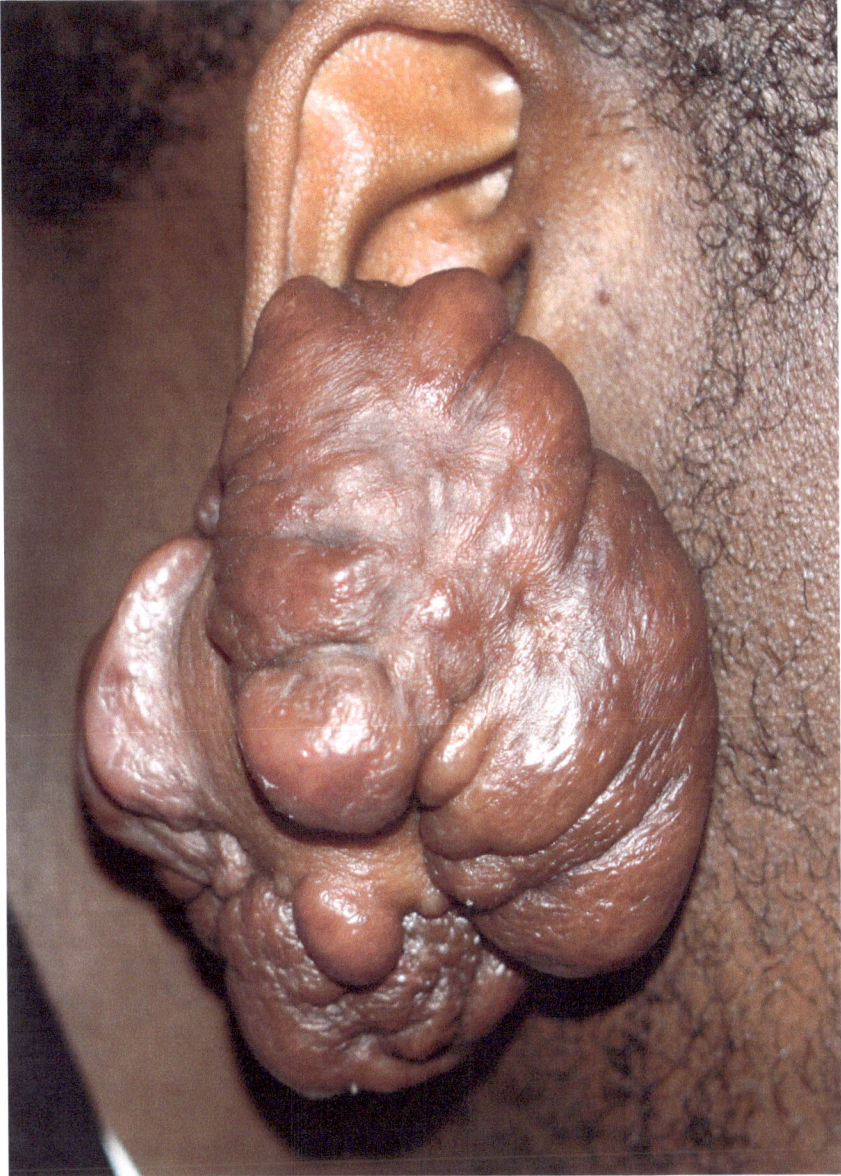

Fig. 86: Very massive ear keloid on right ear. Such keloids, aside from their psycho-social impact, cause certain physical impairments such as being pulled during sleep and causing pain that will wake the patient up, resulting in sleep disturbances. The sheer weight of this keloid was a major problem for this patient.

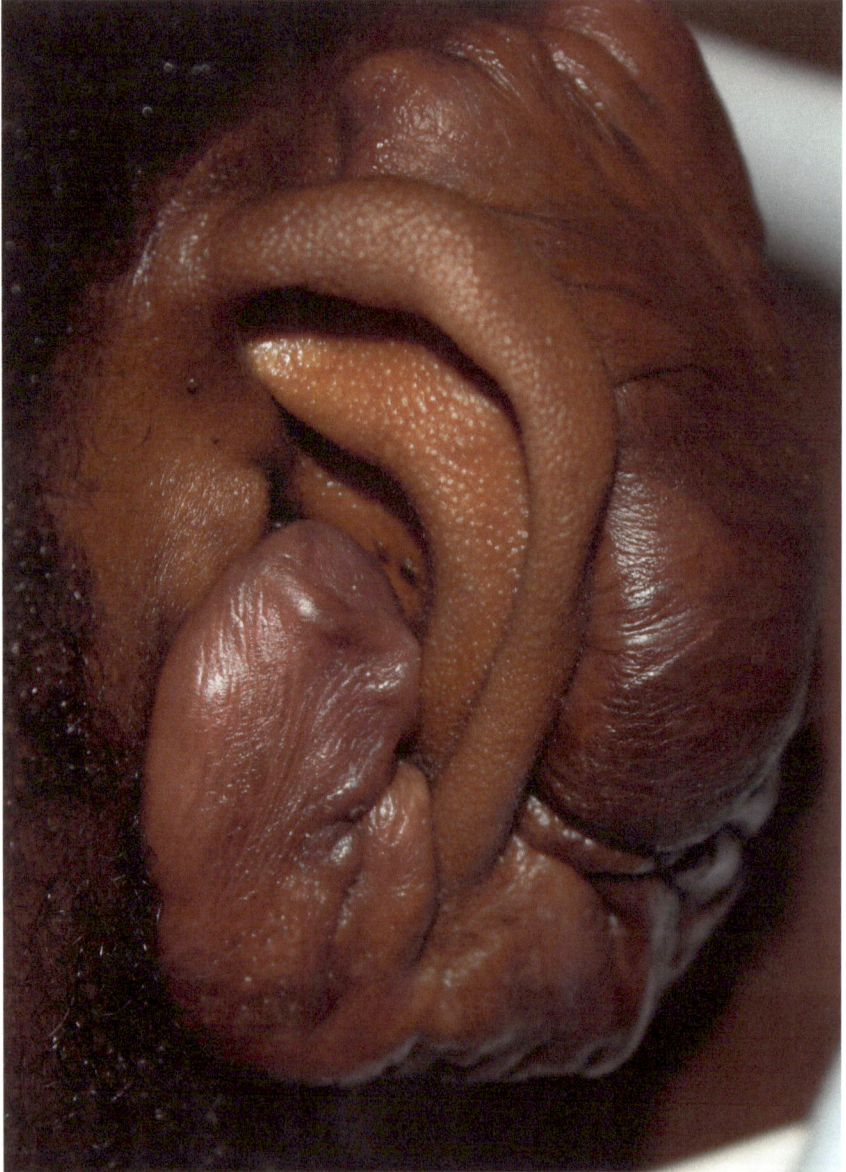

Fig. 87: Massive keloid of left ear in the patient as depicted in *Fig. 86*. Note this keloid has grown inside, and obstructed, the ear canal. This patient had lost his hearing in this ear.

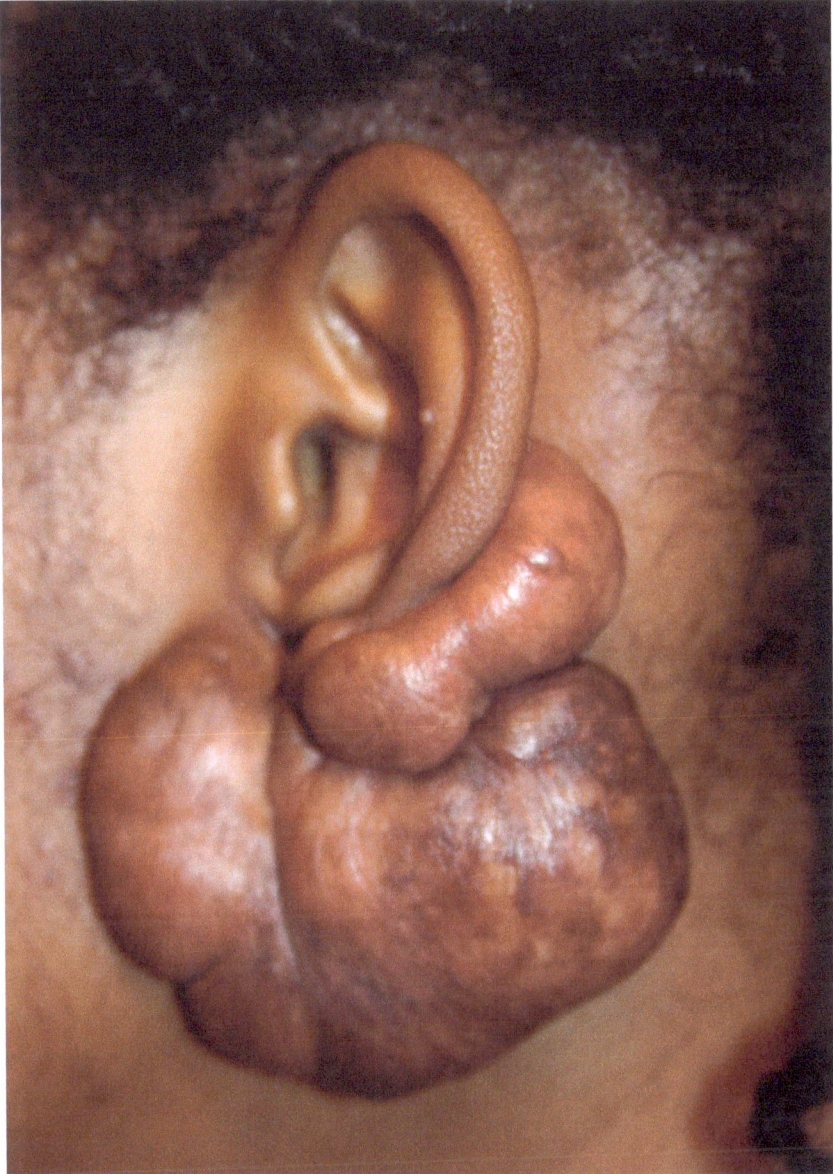

Fig. 88: Massive ear keloid that has spread to the face from the left earlobe area.

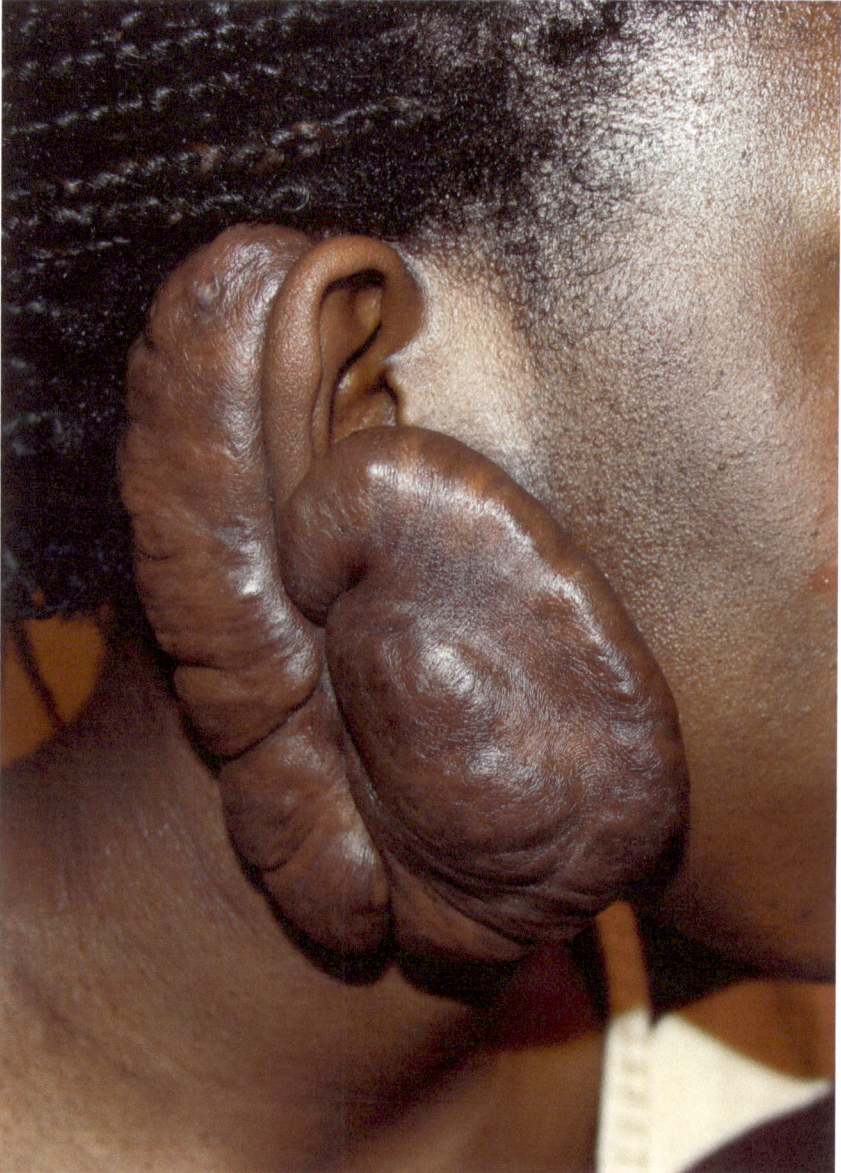

Fig. 89: No words can describe the devastation this keloid has brought to the life of this young woman,

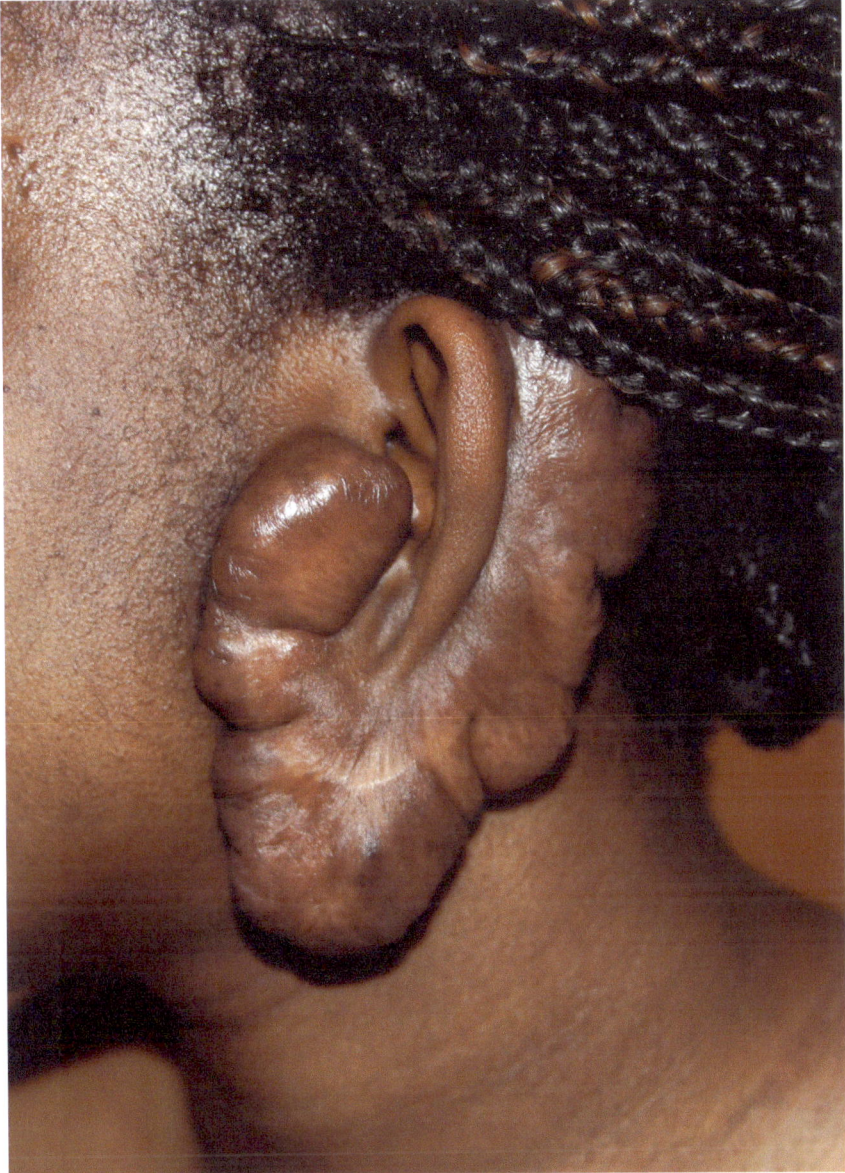

Fig. 90: The same patient as in *Fig. 89*

6 KELOID SPREAD TO FACE

ANOTHER COMPLICATION OF surgery to remove ear keloids is the development of secondary keloids that, due to their more aggressive nature, grow larger and spread outside the boundaries of the ear and onto the face. This is in contrast to primary ear keloids that never spread outside the ear.

The spread of secondary ear keloids to the face should be distinguished from primary facial keloids.

Quite often, primary ear keloids grow outwards and protrude through the skin, causing the formation of a mass of abnormal benign tissue. It appears as if surgery changes the behavior of the primary keloid process and makes it more aggressive; to the point that, in some cases, the newly formed secondary keloids follow a new pattern of spread and infiltrate under the skin without ever protruding through the skin. These keloids form and spread deep under the skin.

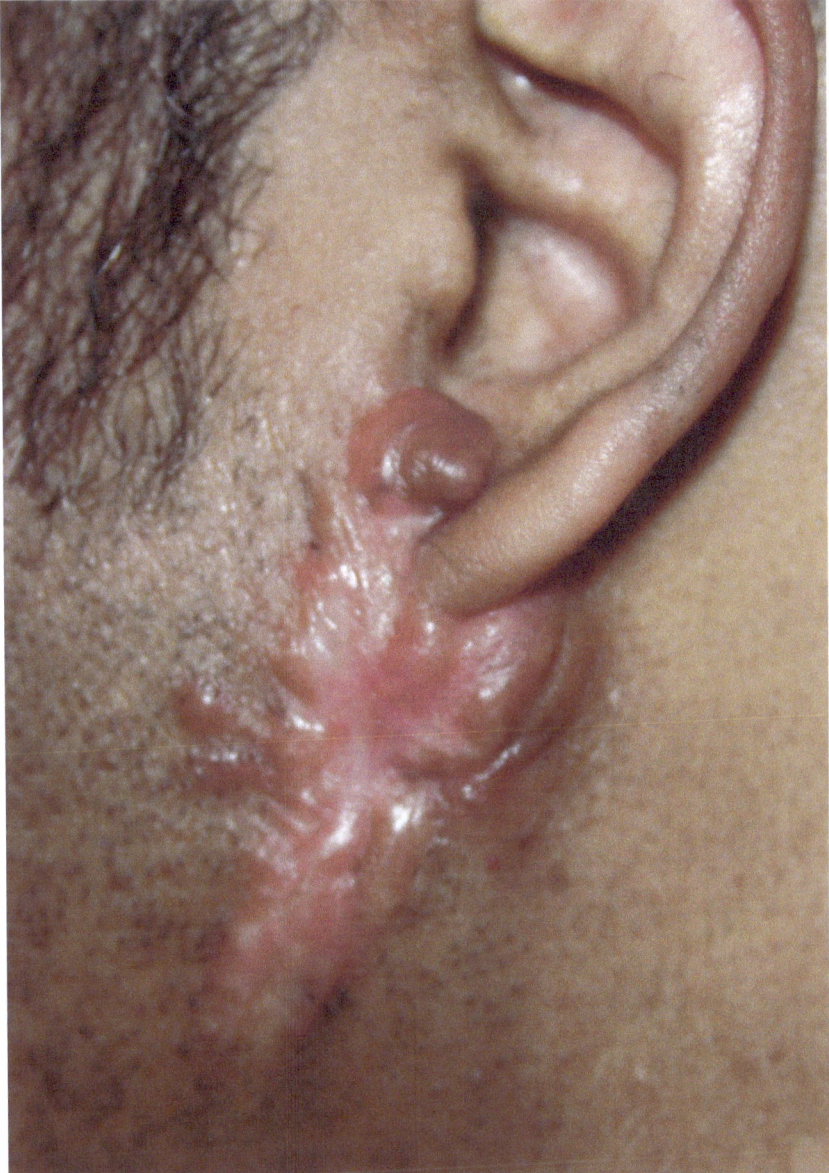

Fig. 91: Secondary ear keloid that has spread to the face from the ear. Note the total absence of the earlobe, which has been removed by prior surgery. The recurrent ear keloid has spread to the face from different directions.

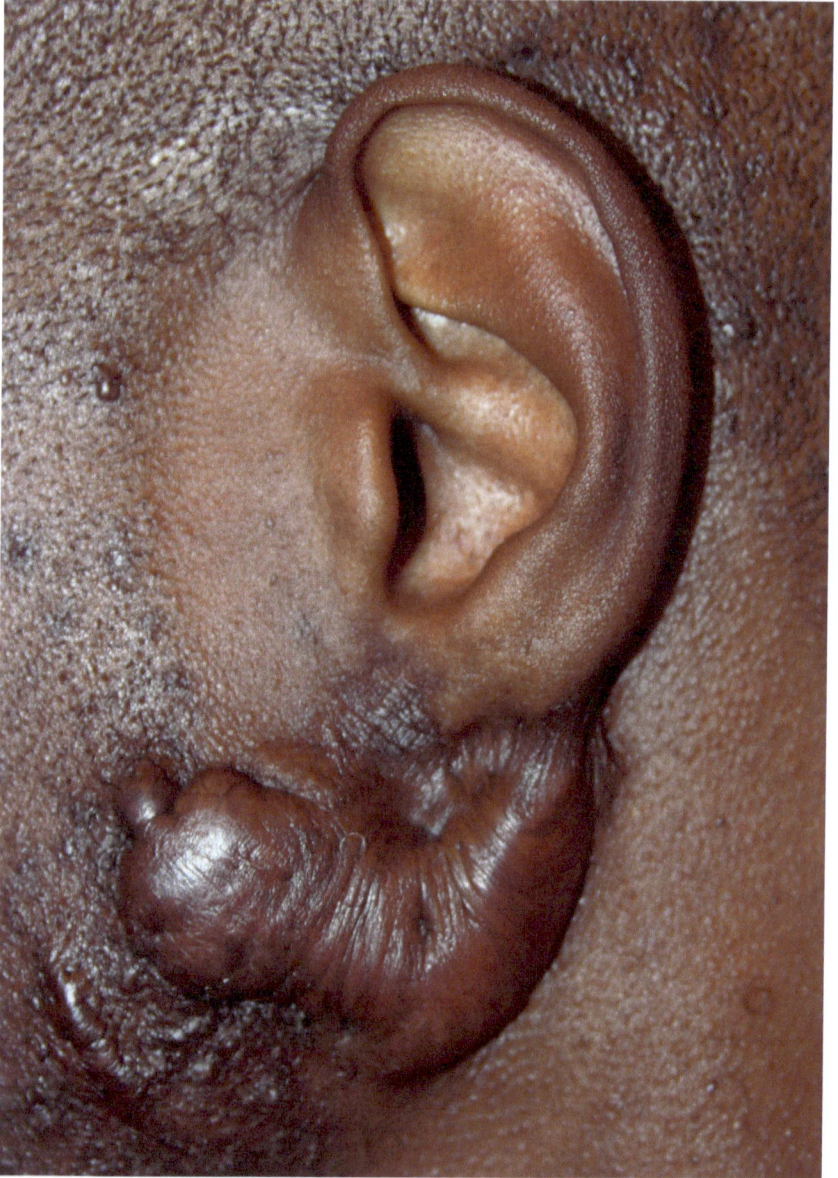

Fig. 92: Secondary ear keloid that has spread to the face from the left ear. Note the total absence of the earlobe, which has been removed by prior surgery. The recurrent ear keloid has spread to the face and merged with prior facial keloids.

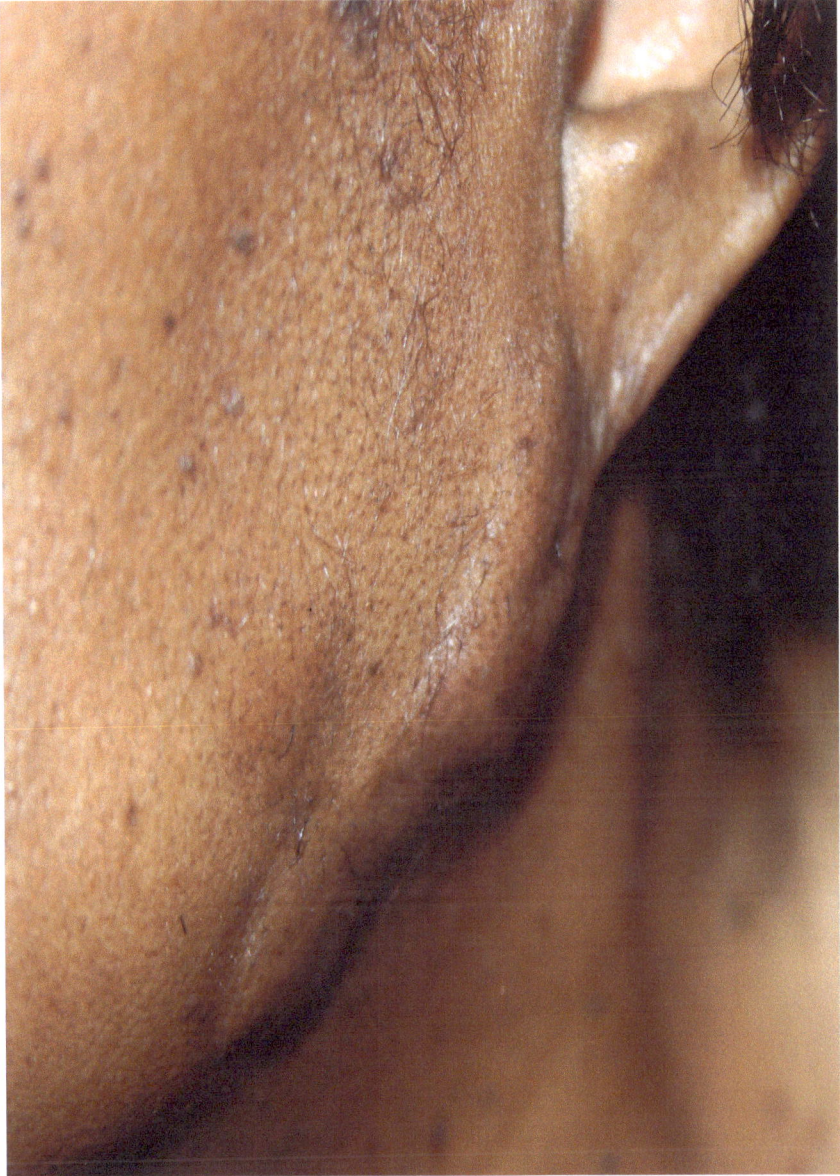

Fig. 93: Secondary ear keloid that has spread to the face from the left earlobe area. Note the total absence of the earlobe, which has been removed by prior surgery. The recurrent keloid process in this case has taken the unique subcutaneous infiltrative pattern, spreading over the mandible.

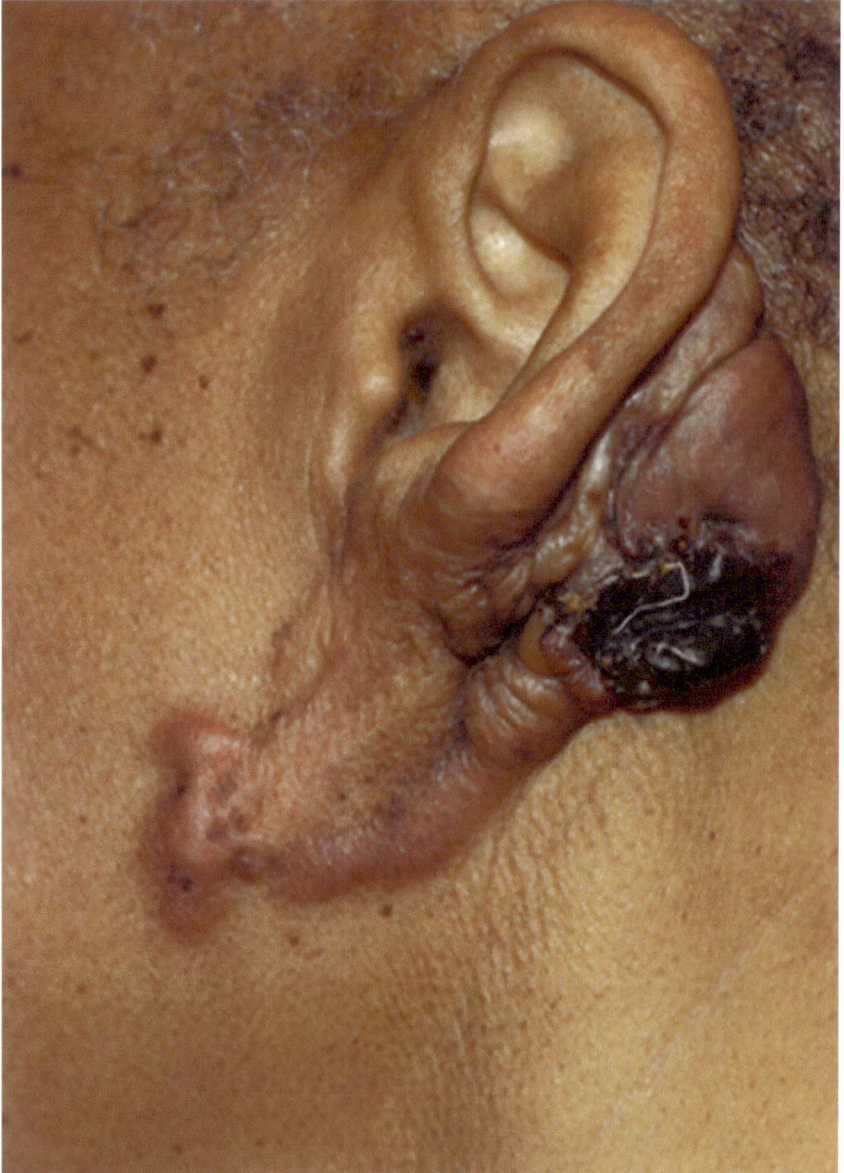

Fig. 94: Secondary ear keloid that has spread to the face from the left earlobe area, as well as over the mastoid bone and behind the ear. Again, note the total absence of the earlobe, which has been removed by prior surgery.

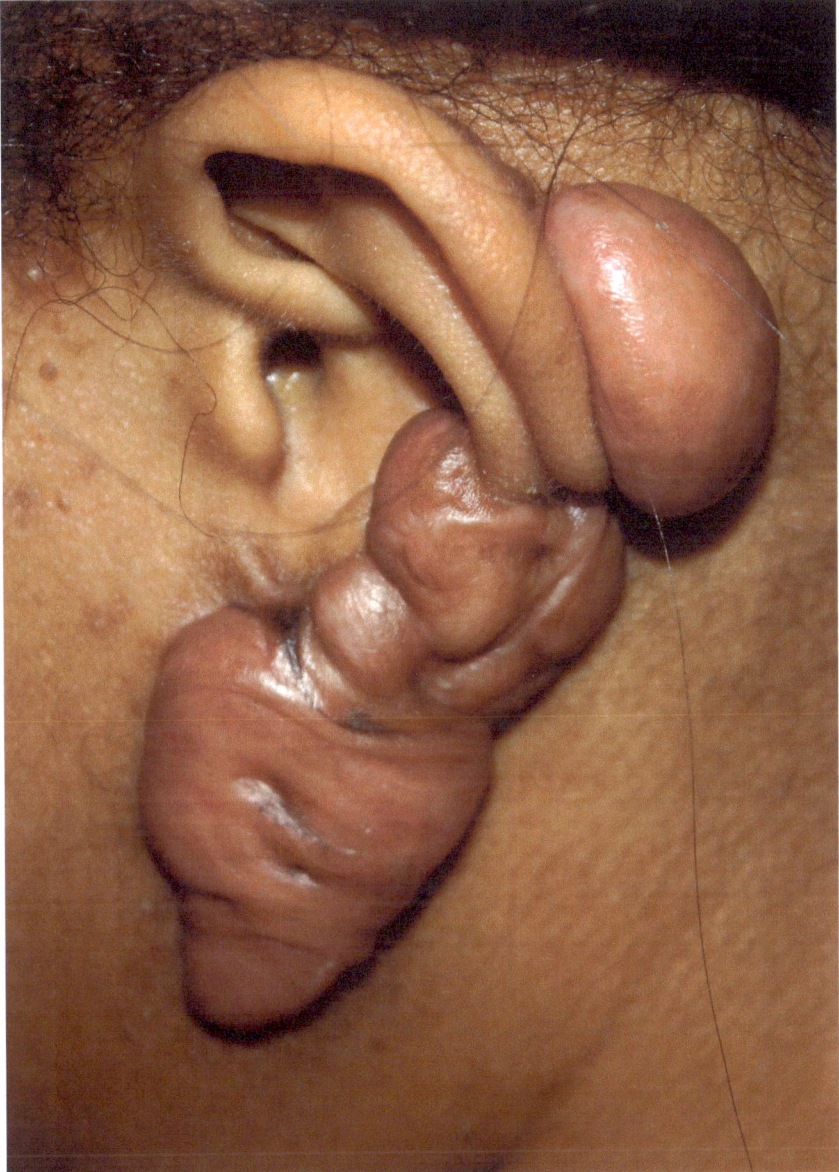

Fig. 95: Secondary ear keloid that has spread to the face from the left earlobe area. Again, note the total absence of the earlobe, which has been removed by prior surgery.

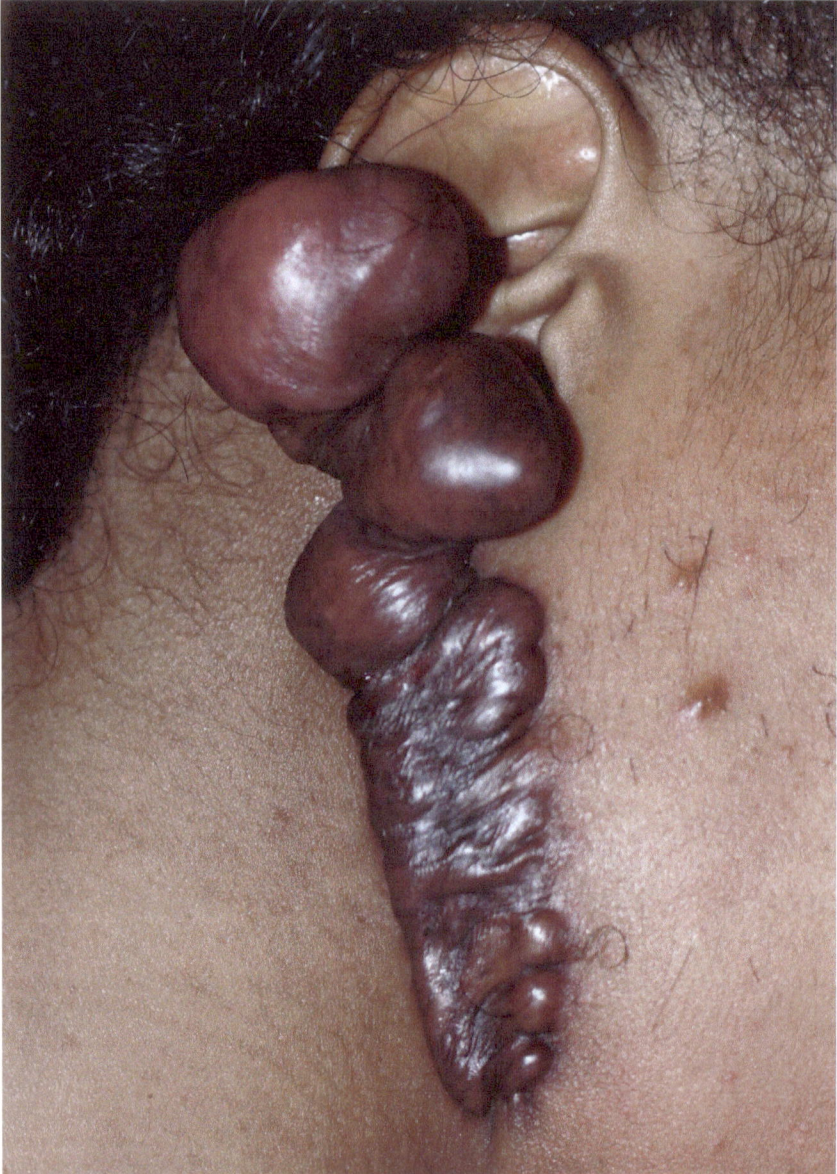

Fig. 96: Secondary ear keloid that has spread to the face from the right earlobe area.

7 EAR KELOIDS AFTER OTOPLASTY

OTOPLASTY IS A surgical procedure employed to revise the shape of or to correct deformities of the external ears.

When performed in individuals who are genetically prone to develop keloids, surgery can lead to the formation of keloidal tumor masses. These keloids can grow to become very large. The size of primary otoplasty keloids is directly tied to the time elapsed since otoplasty.

Over the years, the author has treated ten patients with this condition. Most patients have an Eastern European background and eight were male. All ten patients were Caucasians. The author has not seen a single case of post-otoplasty keloid among African Americans; perhaps the procedure does not have much utility among African Americans.

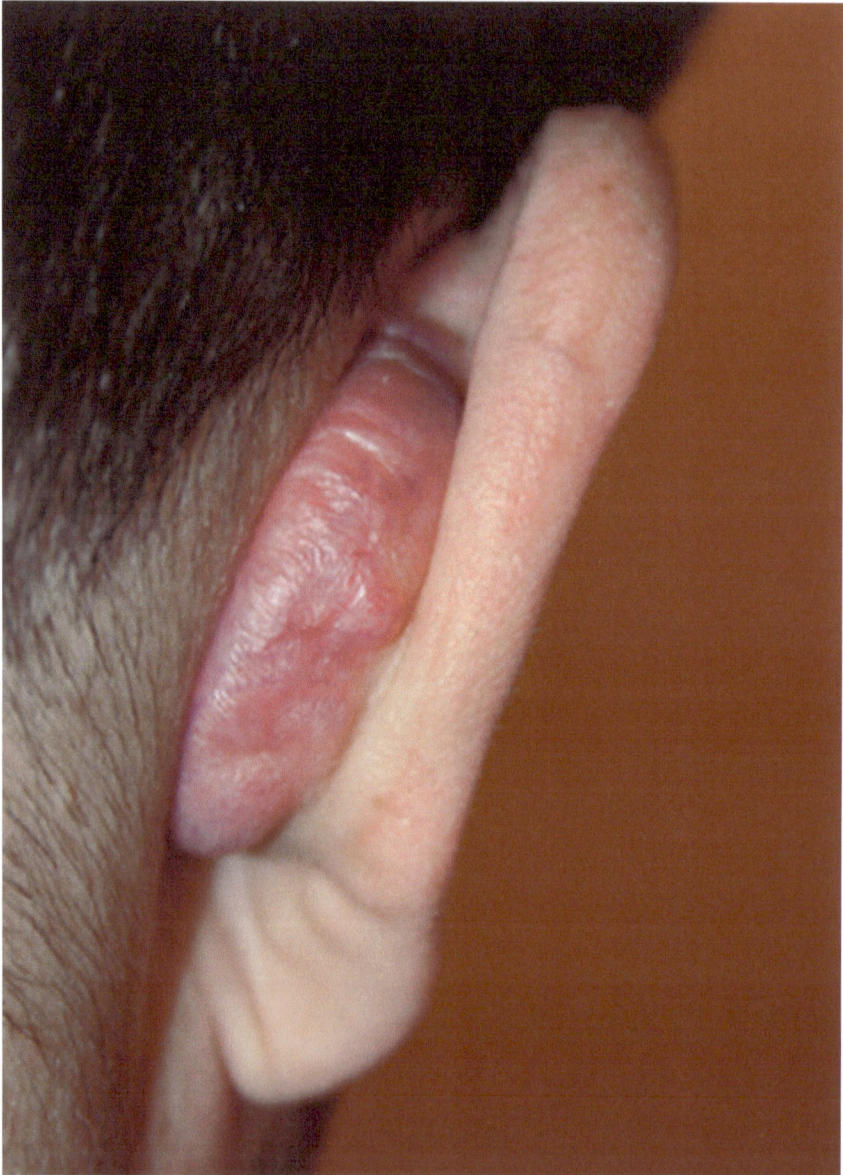

Fig. 97: Otoplasty keloid of right ear.

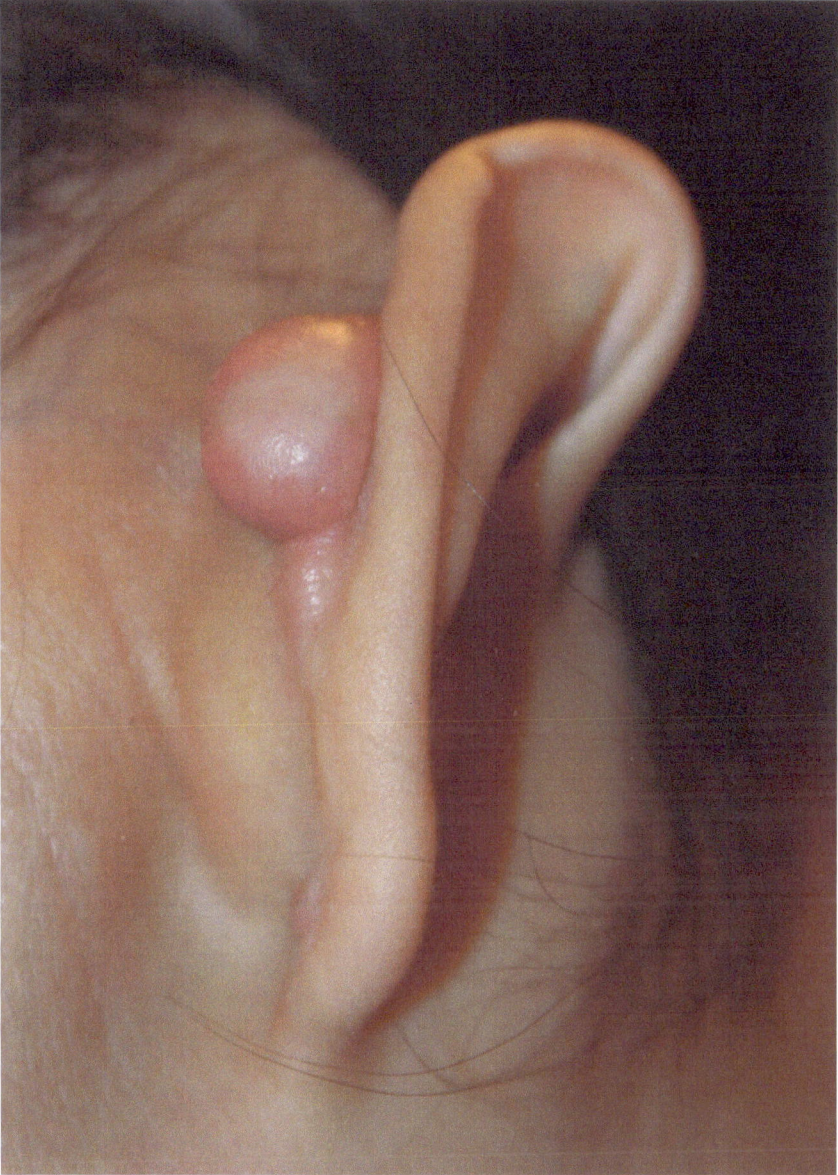

Fig. 98: Otoplasty keloid of right ear.

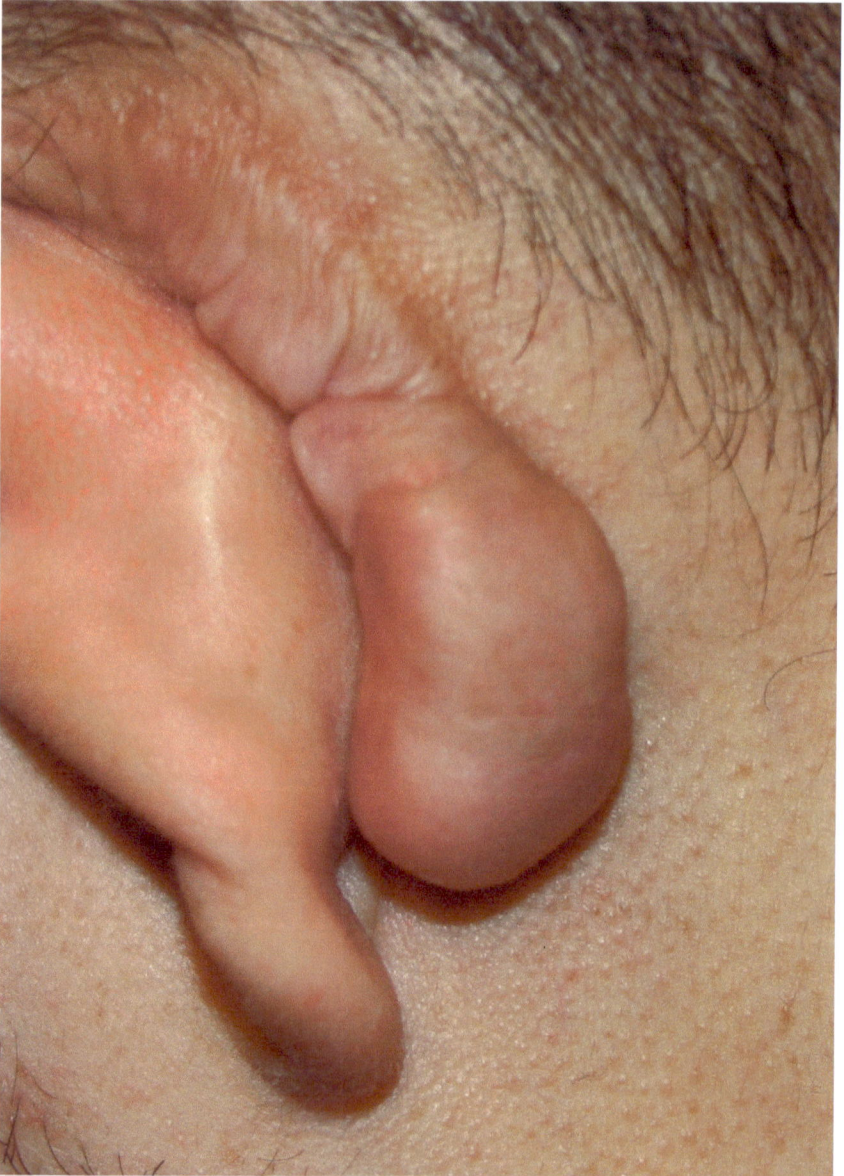

Fig. 99: Otoplasty keloid of left ear.

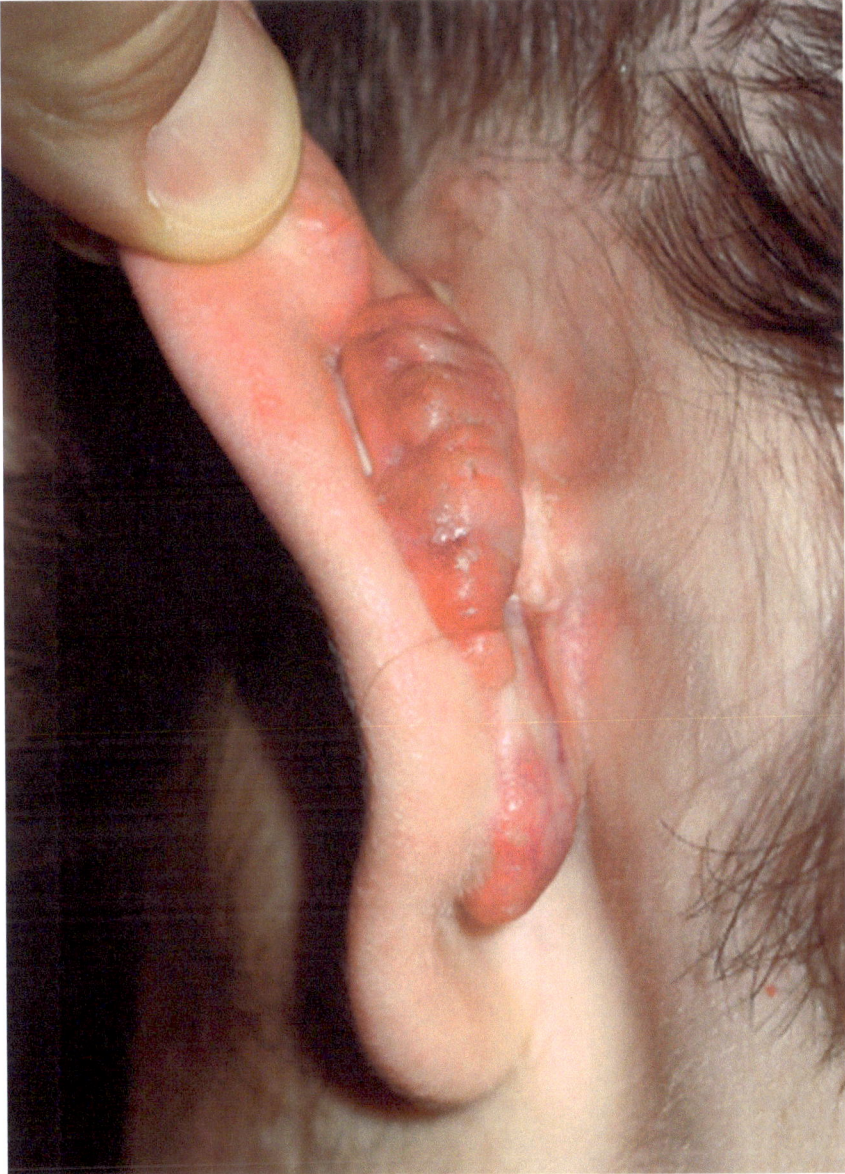

Fig. 100: Otoplasty keloid of left ear.

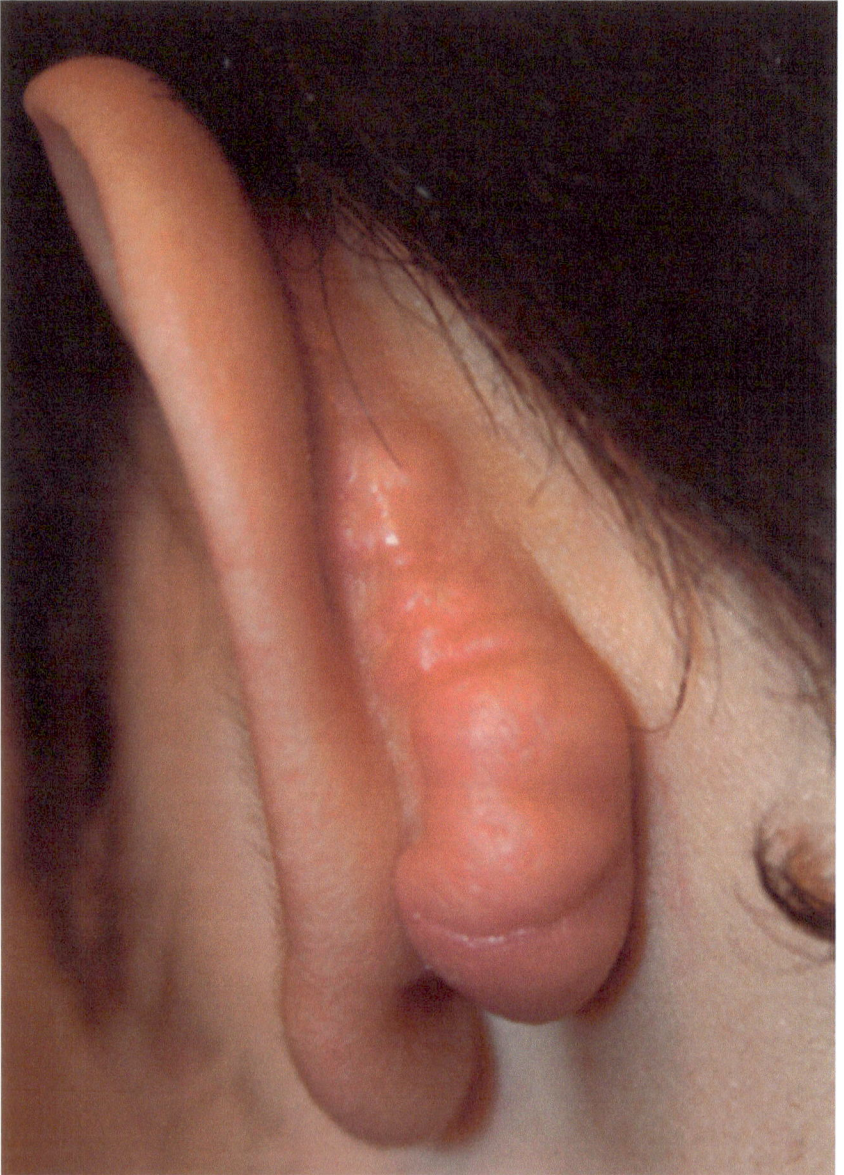

Fig. 101: Otoplasty keloid of left ear.

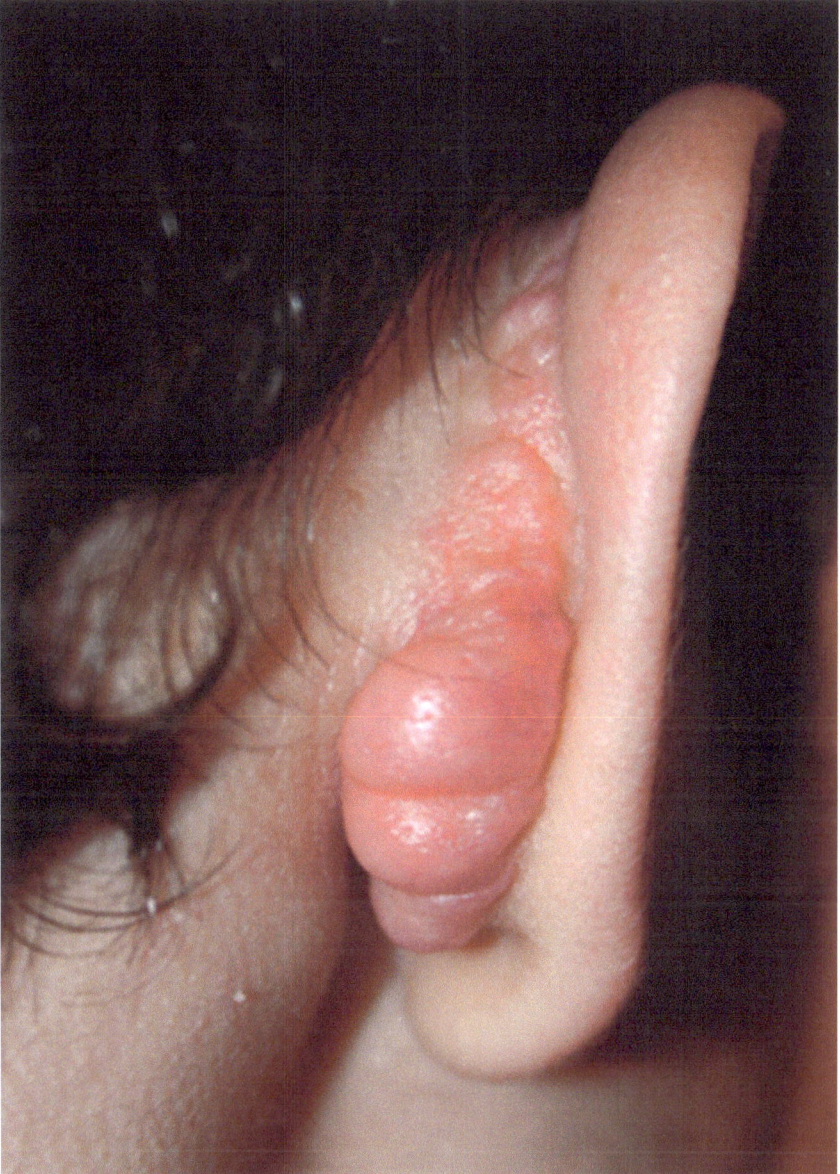

Fig. 102: Otoplasty keloid of right ear in patient shown in *Fig 101*.

8 EAR KELOIDS AFTER FACELIFT SURGERY

FACELIFT SURGERY IS a common esthetic procedure performed to enhance the appearance of the face and to reduce wrinkles. The standard facelift procedure involves several incisions that usually start in the hair or hairline above and in front of each ear and extend below the ears, and around the earlobes, continuing upwards behind the ears. During this procedure, the surgeon removes excess facial skin from this area and then closes the wound.

Oftentimes, the wounds heal well and the esthetic outcome of the procedure is very satisfactory. However; when the procedure is performed in individuals who are genetically prone to developing keloids, the wounds will not heal normally and result in the formation of keloid lesions. The size and location of facelift keloids varies from patient to patient, and is most likely related to the severity of the genetic propensity to develop keloids.

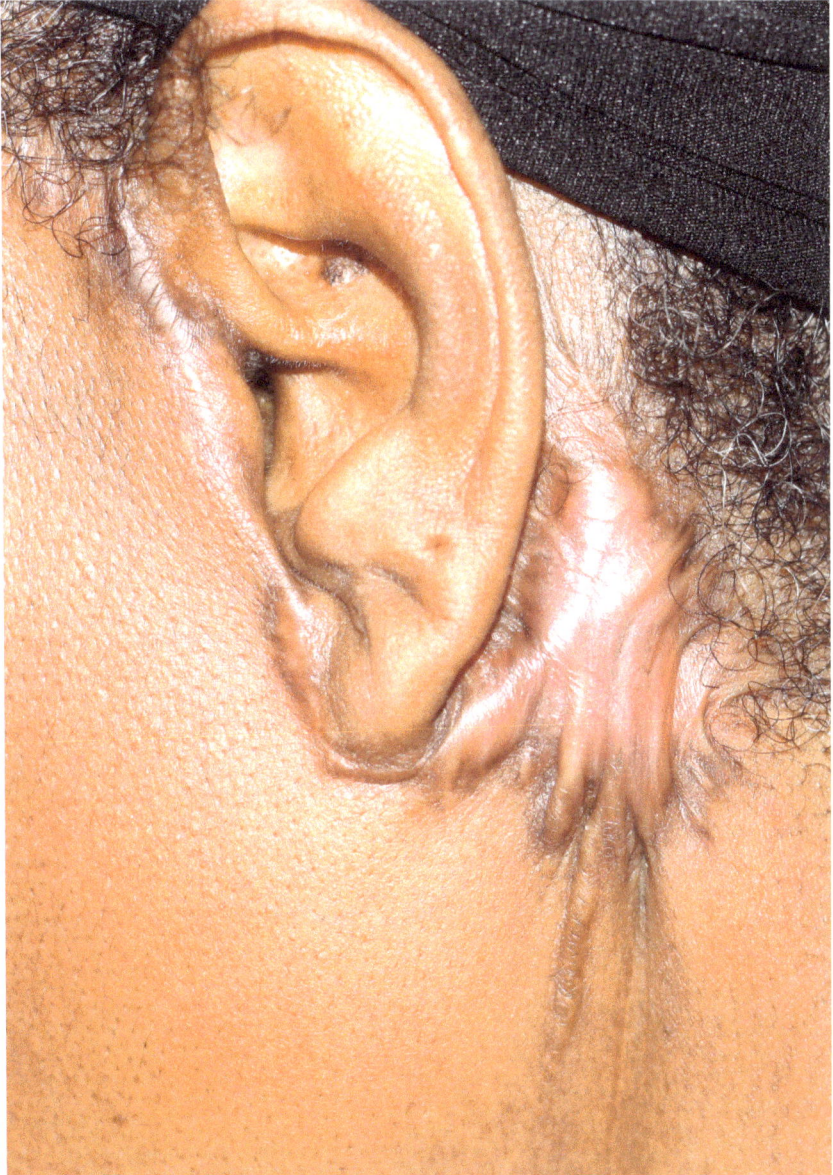

Fig. 103: Keloid formation near and around the left ear from a facelift procedure.

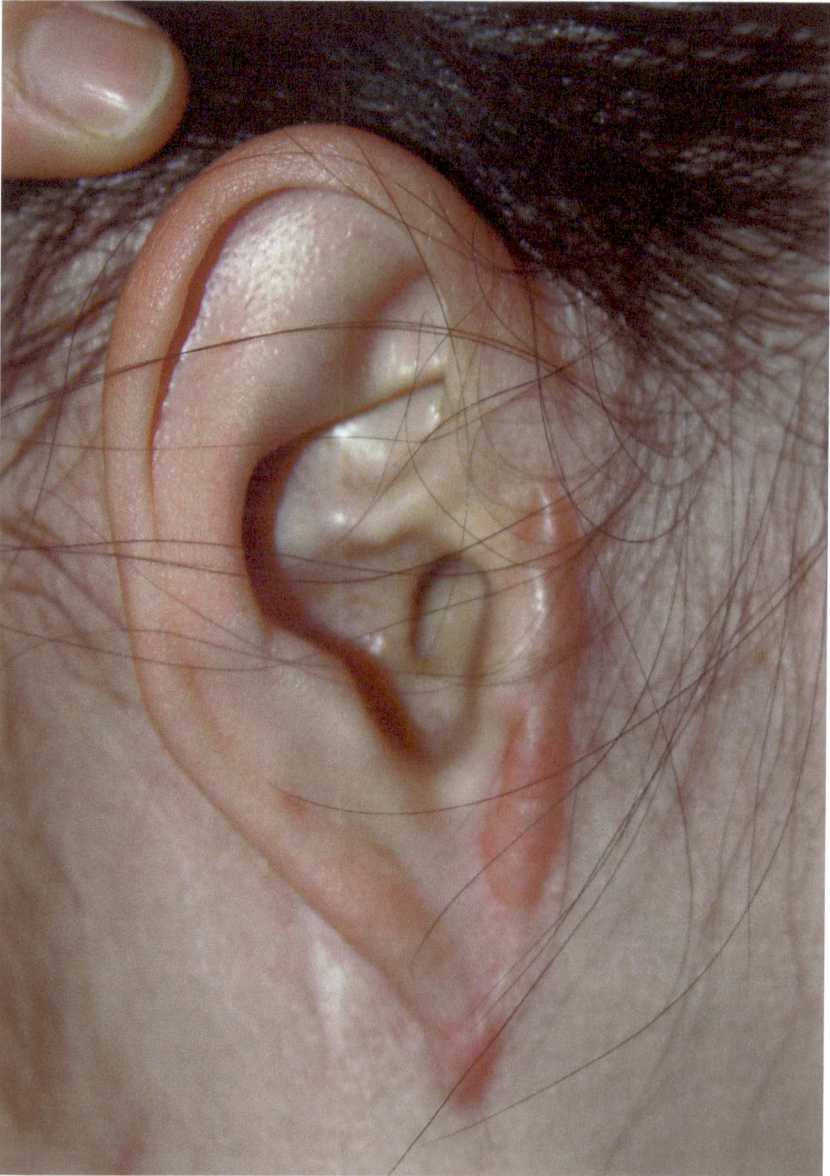

Fig. 104: Keloid formation from a facelift procedure, right ear.

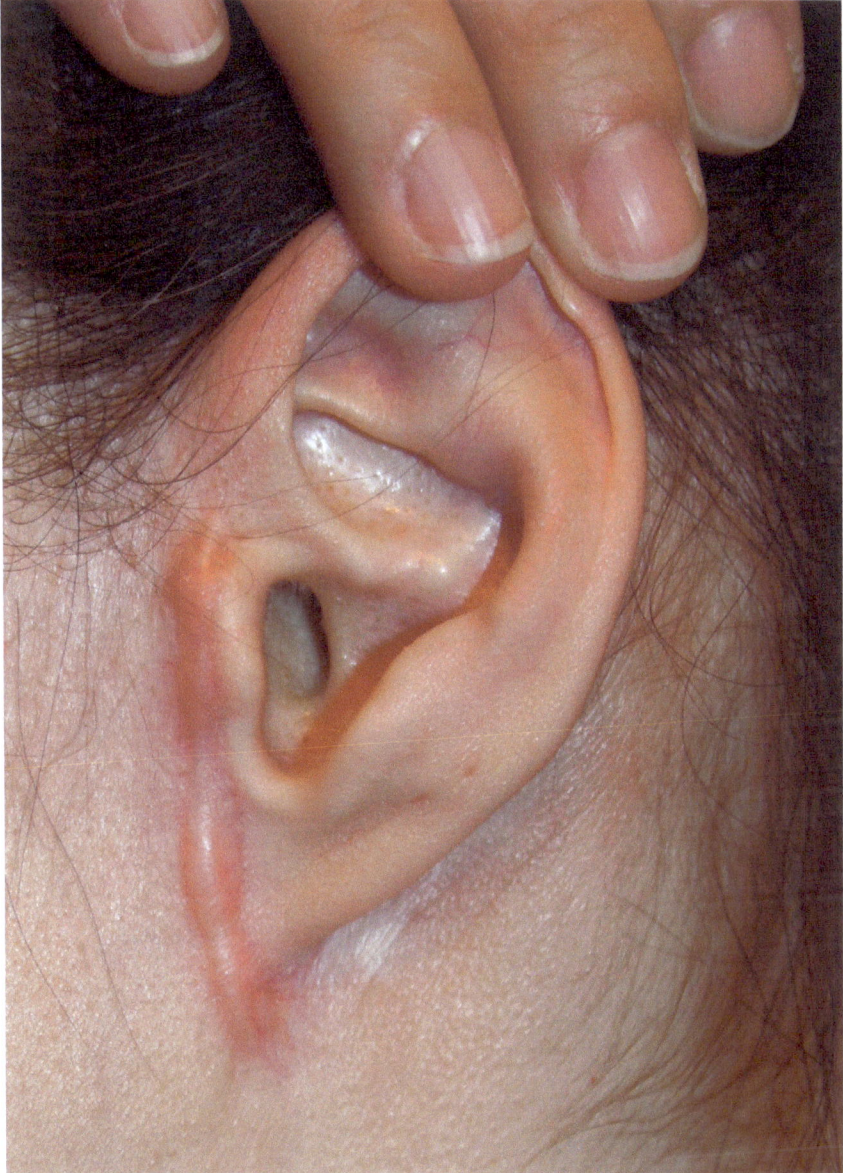

Fig. 105: Keloid formation from a facelift procedure, left ear of the same patient shown in *Fig 104*

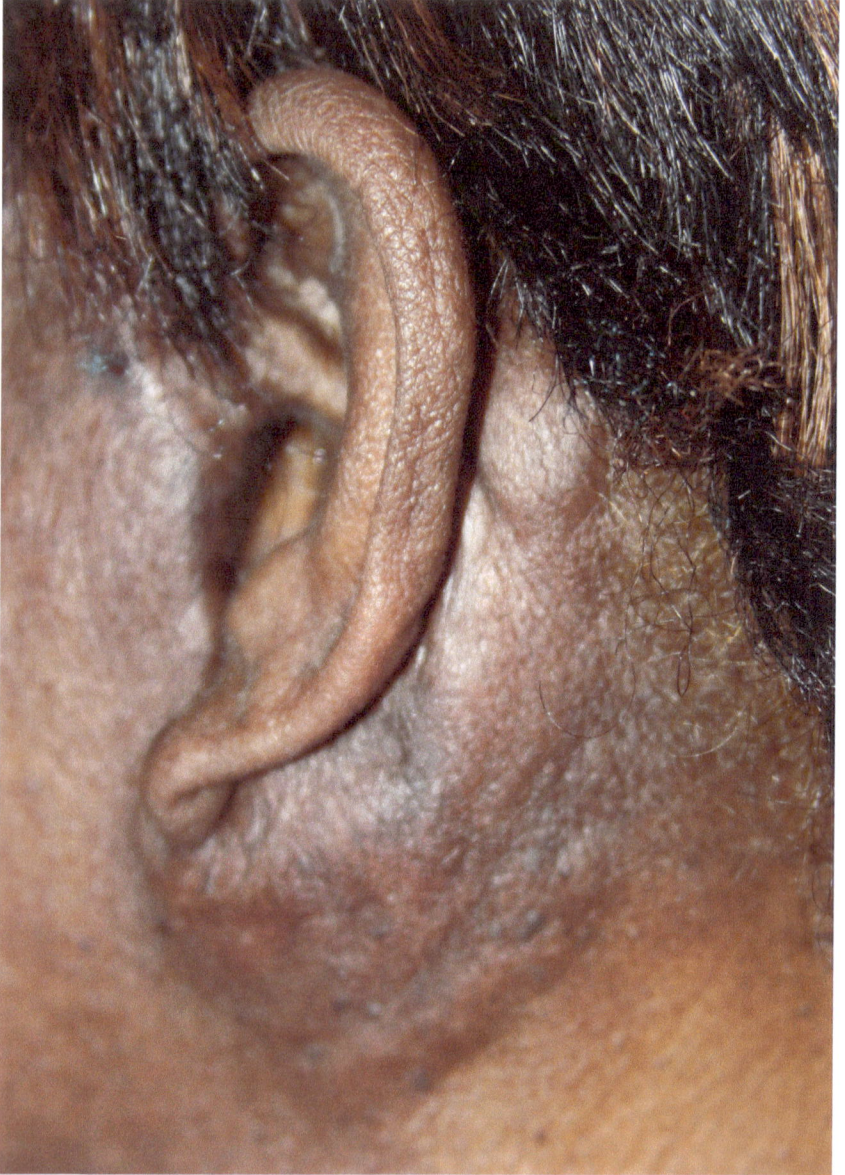

Fig. 106: Peri-auricular infiltrative keloid formation from a facelift procedure, left ear.

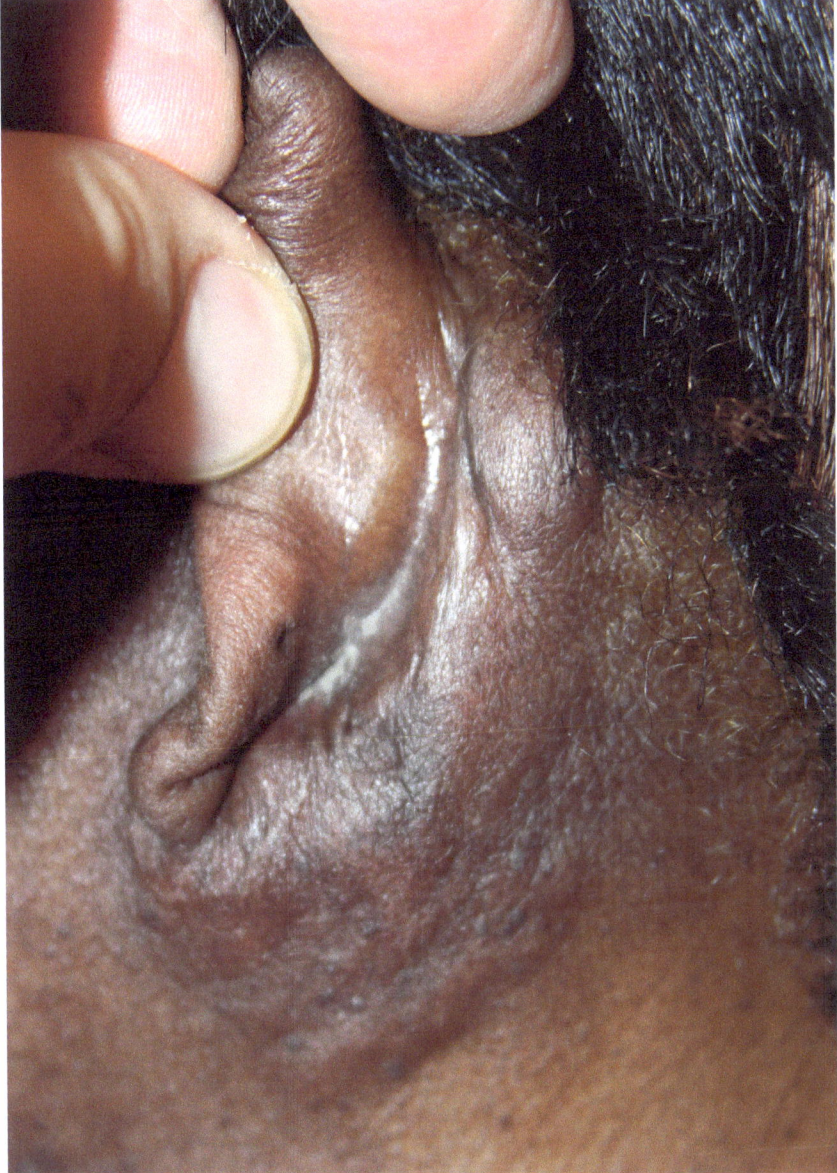

Fig. 107: Peri-auricular infiltrative keloid formation from a facelift procedure, left ear, same patient as shown in *Fig. 106*

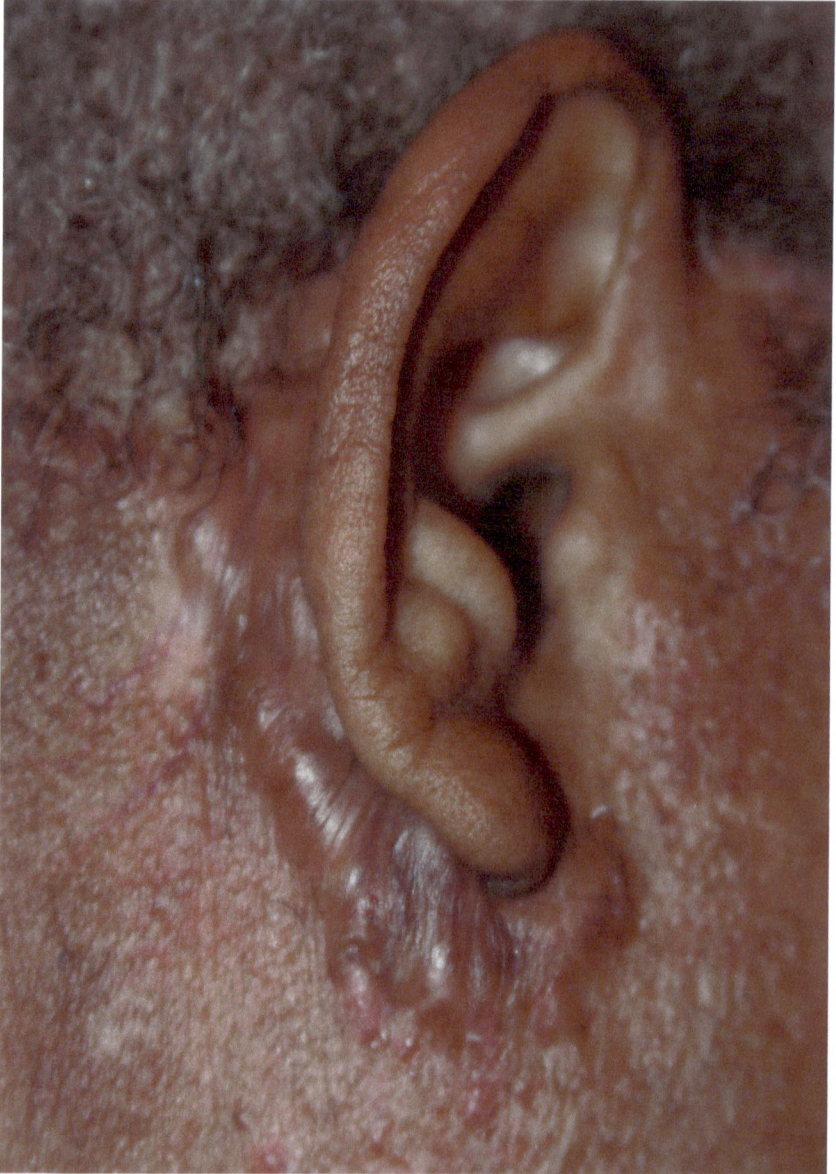

Fig. 108: Keloid formation from a facelift procedure, right ear.

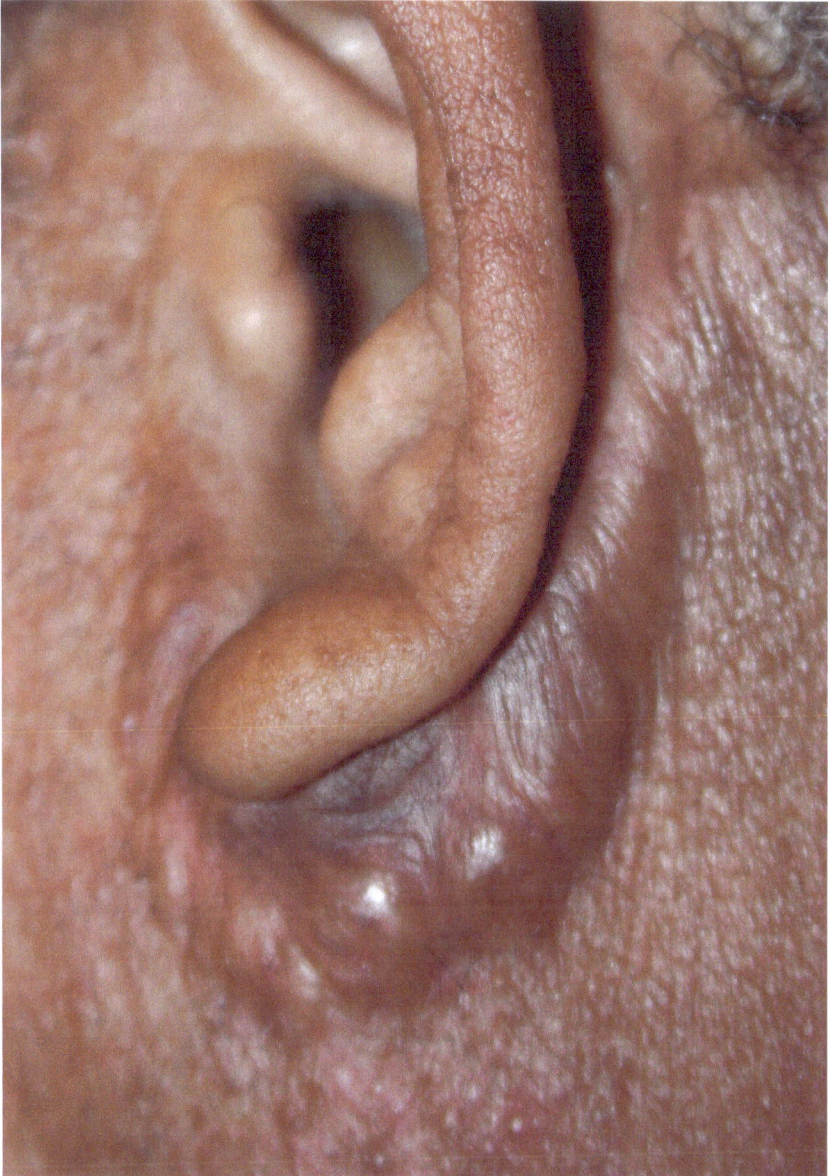

Fig. 109: Keloid formation from a facelift procedure, left ear, same patient as shown in *Fig 108*.

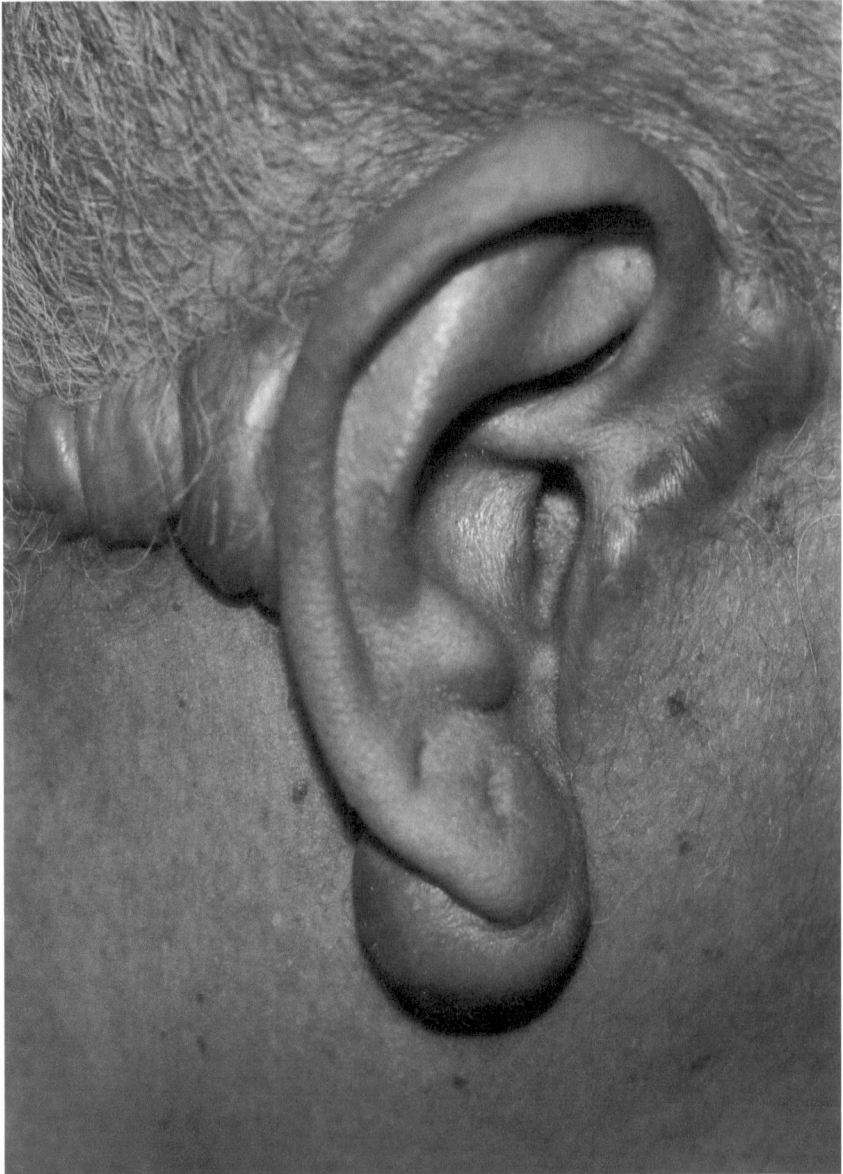

Fig. 110: Keloid formation from a facelift procedure, right ear. Notice the nodular keloid formation below the right earlobe.

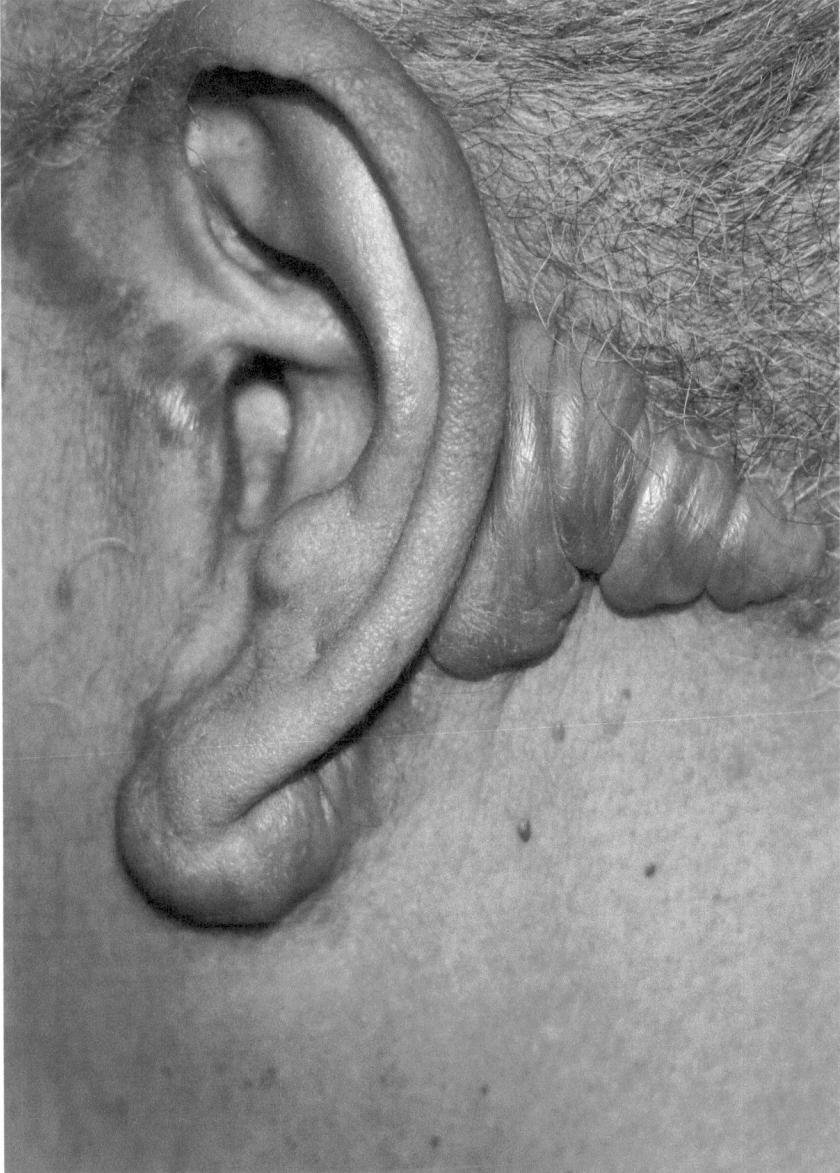

Fig. 111: Keloid formation from a facelift procedure, right ear, same patient shown in *Fig. 110*.

9 CRYOTHERAPY

THE SUCCESSFUL TREATMENT of human diseases is reliant on a thorough understanding of the underlying processes that lead to the development of particular illnesses. The treatment of diabetes with insulin or of bacterial infections with antibiotics are good examples of this scientific methodology. Unfortunately, when it comes to keloid, the lack of basic understanding of the disease process often leads to unsatisfactory therapeutic results.

The basic principal of treating keloidal lesions is the destruction of the abnormal tissue with a method that will not trigger the wound healing response. The surgical removal of keloids will, indeed, trigger the underlying pathological wound healing response and, therefore, result in a worsening of keloids; not to mention the detrimental loss of normal ear tissue from surgery.

All primary ear keloids can be successfully treated with non-surgical methods, with significantly better esthetic outcomes. This approach, however, takes time and requires patience and proper planning.

The systematic following of this approach by all healthcare providers will most definitely prevent the development of incurable secondary keloids.

Treatment of Primary Ear Keloids

The best treatment approach for very small ear keloids is cryotherapy for all lesions that protrude from the skin, with or without intra-lesional steroid injections for lesions that reside within the body of ear tissue. The biggest mistake in treating primary ear keloids is to go after the core of the keloid that resides within the ear tissue with a surgical scalpel. The core of the keloid should only be treated with intra-lesional steroids or pressure devices.

Cryotherapy should be (1) delivered properly and (2) repeated as many times to the keloid as needed. The simple spraying of liquid nitrogen to the surface of keloid with a handheld spray gun is not considered proper cryotherapy. Liquid nitrogen is best applied with a small applicator, such as a cotton swab, dipped in liquid nitrogen and applied to the keloid with gentle pressure. This process should be repeated until the whole mass of keloid is frozen to the level of normal ear tissue.

Cryotherapy remains the best treatment option for almost all primary ear keloids and works very well for almost everyone. Most ear keloids need an average of three rounds of treatments, given once every six to eight weeks.

As opposed to surgery, proper application of cryotherapy does not result in damage to normal ear tissue and does not trigger wound healing response. Within a few hours, treated tissue becomes edematous and swollen, which often transforms to a blister within the first 24 hours. The size of the blister depends upon the size of the primary keloid. Blisters may break and ooze serous fluid for several days to a week. During this time frame, the treated keloid should be attended to as an open wound, and is best covered with a gauze and loose dressing.

Within a week, the treated tissue starts to dry out and forms a dark or black-colored scab which will remain in place until the tissue underneath heals and new epithelium is formed. The scab will then gradually slough off. This process takes as long as three weeks for very small keloids and as long as six to eight weeks for larger keloids. Upon recovery from the first treatment, most keloids lose between thirty and sixty percent of their mass.

Cryotherapy should be repeated at this time and in the same fashion every four to eight weeks, until the mass of keloid is totally destroyed. Depending on the size of the primary keloid, this process often takes four to eight months and results in total removal of the primary keloids in almost every patient. Compliance with this treatment and pain control are essential.

Once the bulk of the keloid is removed, pressure devices or intra-lesional steroids should be used in all those who continue to have a keloid remnant in their ear.

Close clinical monitoring is essential once the keloid is totally removed with cryotherapy. Any recurrences after cryotherapy should be treated as soon as possible and in the same manner. Intra-lesional chemotherapy should be considered for resistant recurrences.

The rate of recurrence of primary ear keloid after cryotherapy is generally low. It is lowest for those who have only one ear keloid and who do not have keloids elsewhere.

A strong family history of keloids, as well as the presence of keloids in other parts of the skin, indicates to a more aggressive nature of the underlying disorder, and is associated with a higher risk of recurrence.

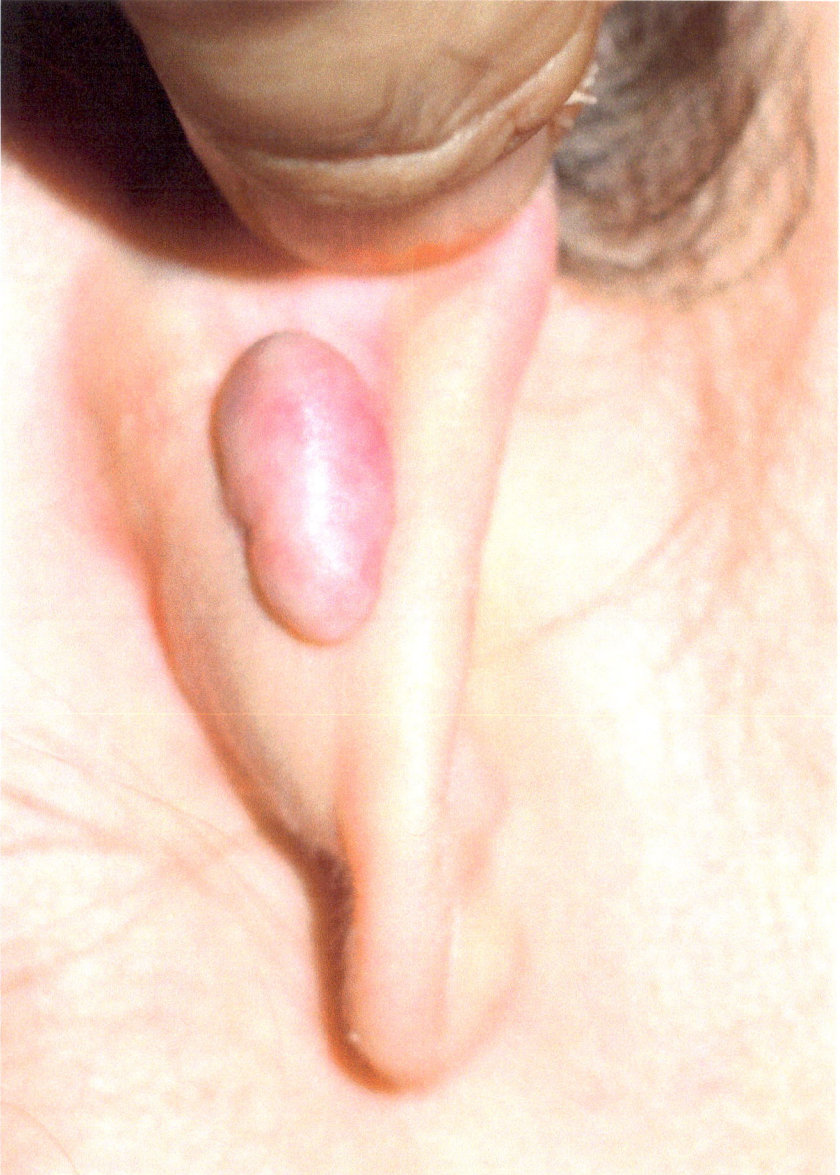

Fig. 112: Primary ear keloid

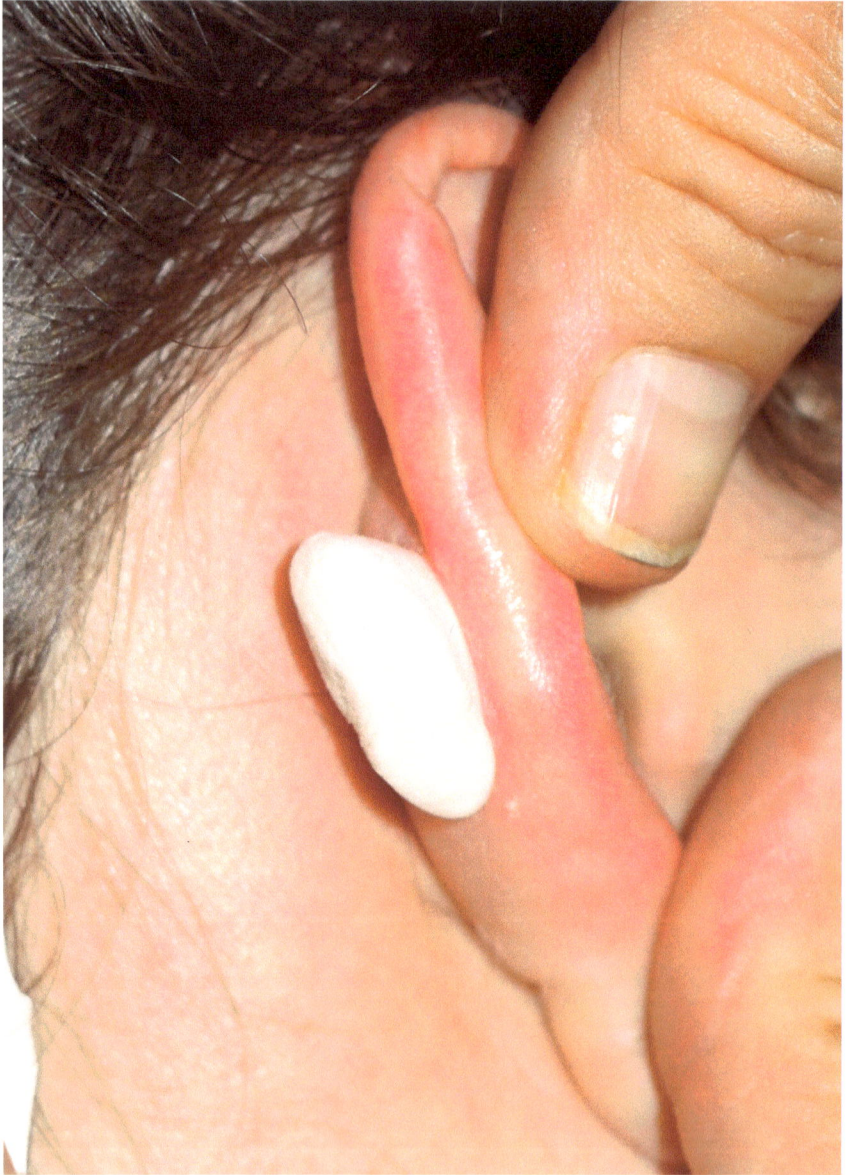

Fig. 113: Primary ear keloid, same patient as shown in *Fig 112*. Immediately after application of cryotherapy. The frozen keloid appears white.

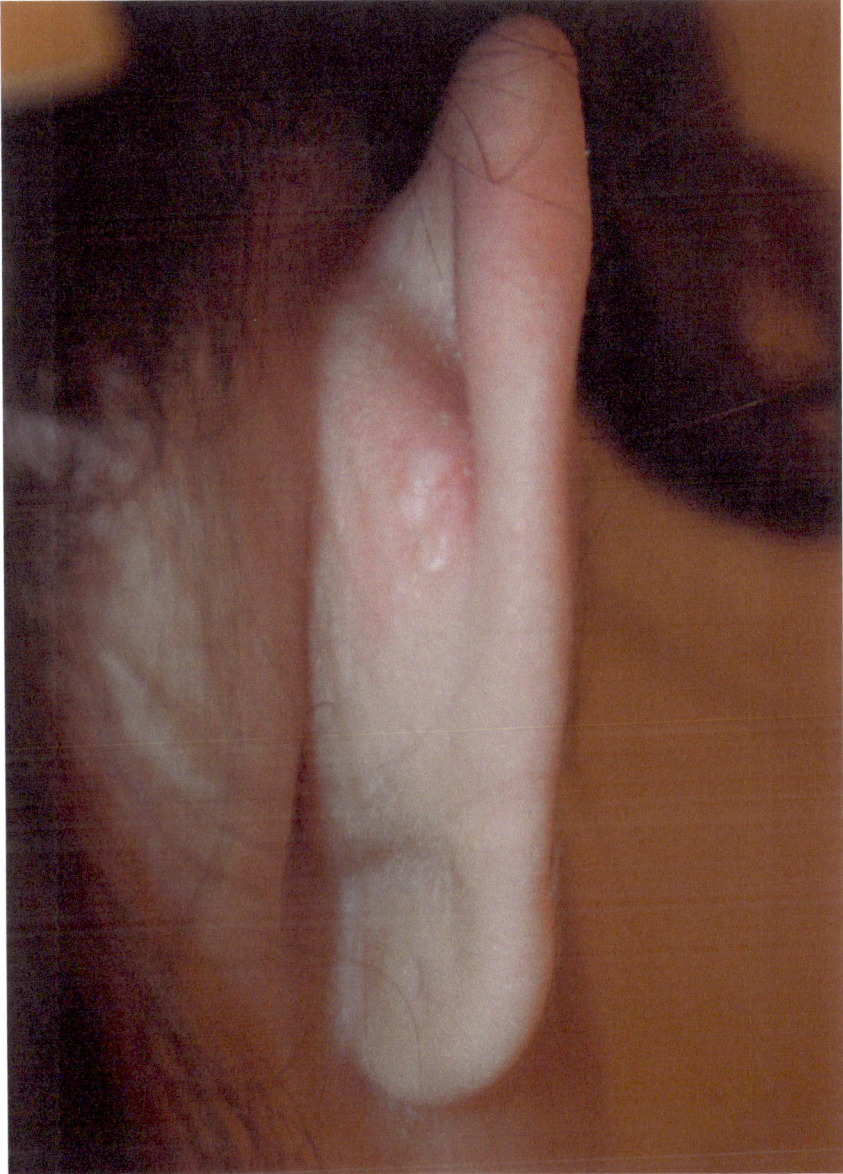

Fig. 114: Primary ear keloid, same patient as shown in *Fig 112* and *113*, three years later.

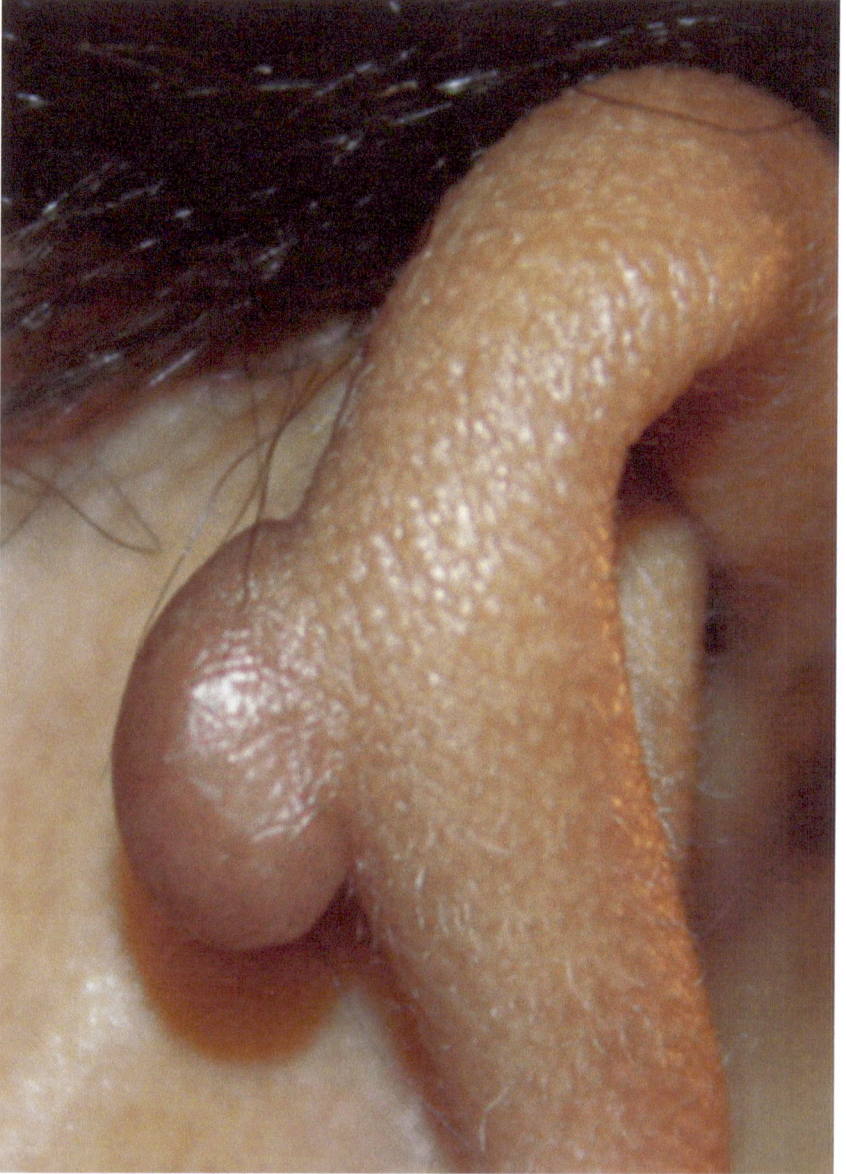

Fig. 115: Primary ear keloid

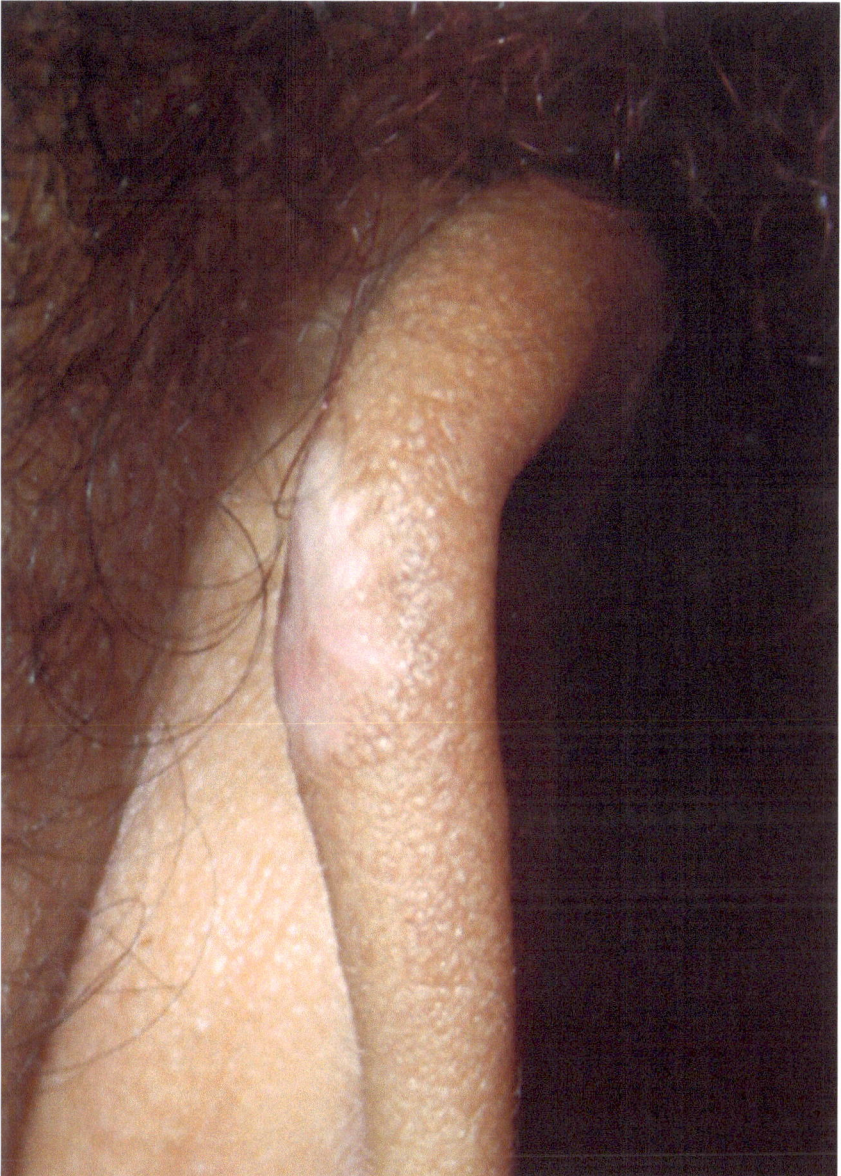

Fig. 116: Same patient as shown in *Fig 115*, one-year follow up after cryotherapy.

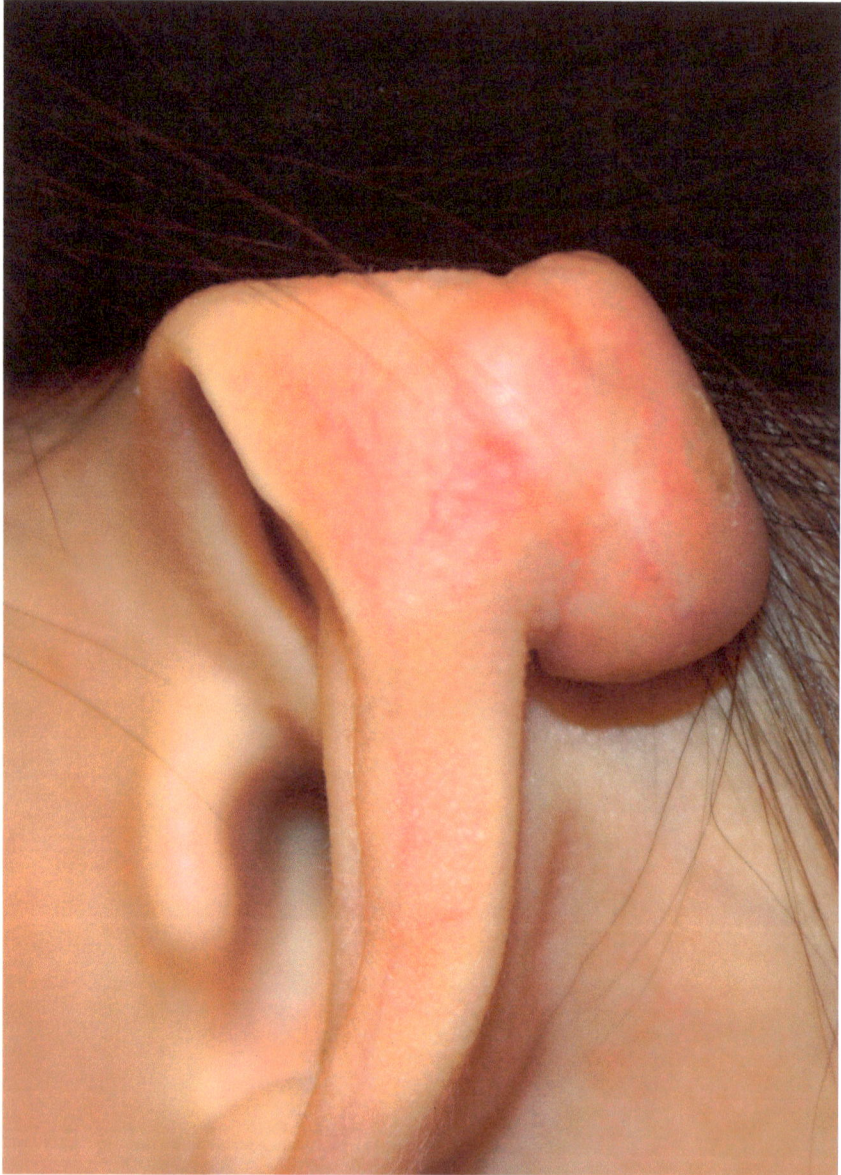

Fig. 117: Primary ear keloid

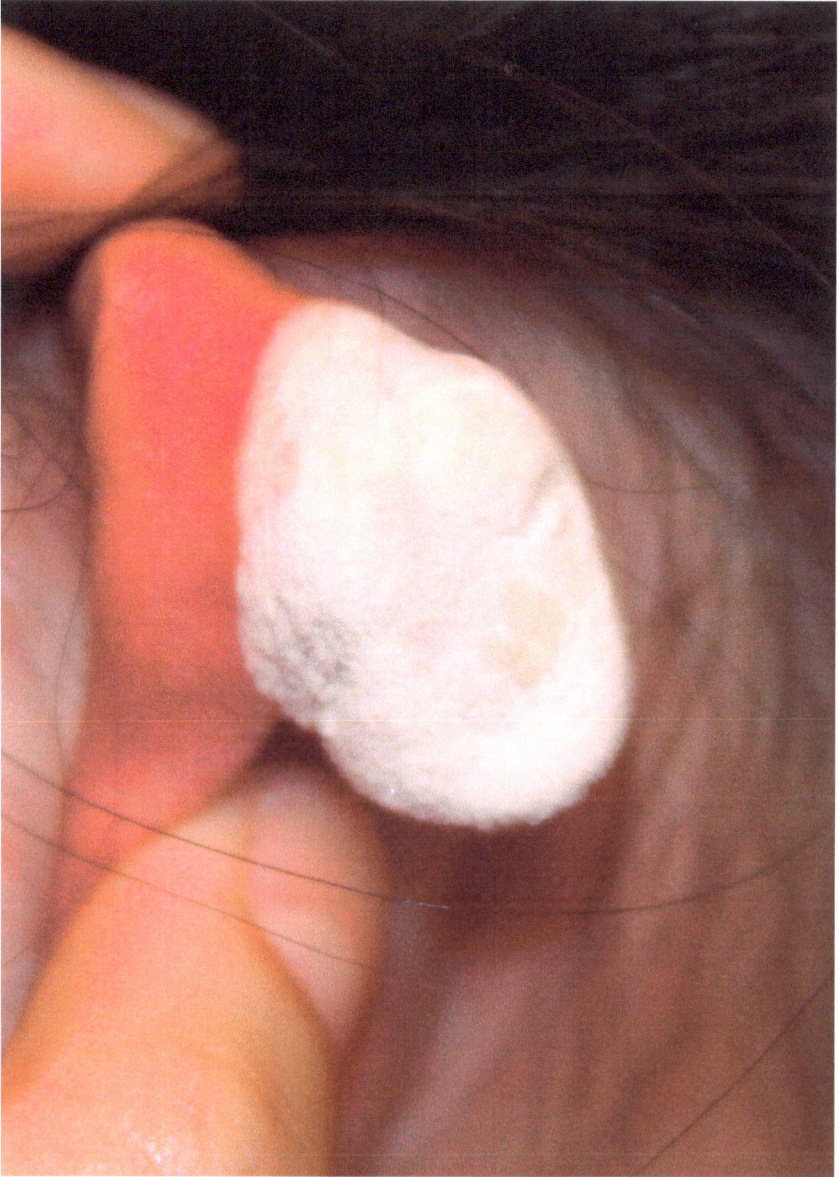

Fig. 118: Primary ear keloid, same patient as shown in *Fig 117*, immediately after application of cryotherapy. The frozen keloid appears white.

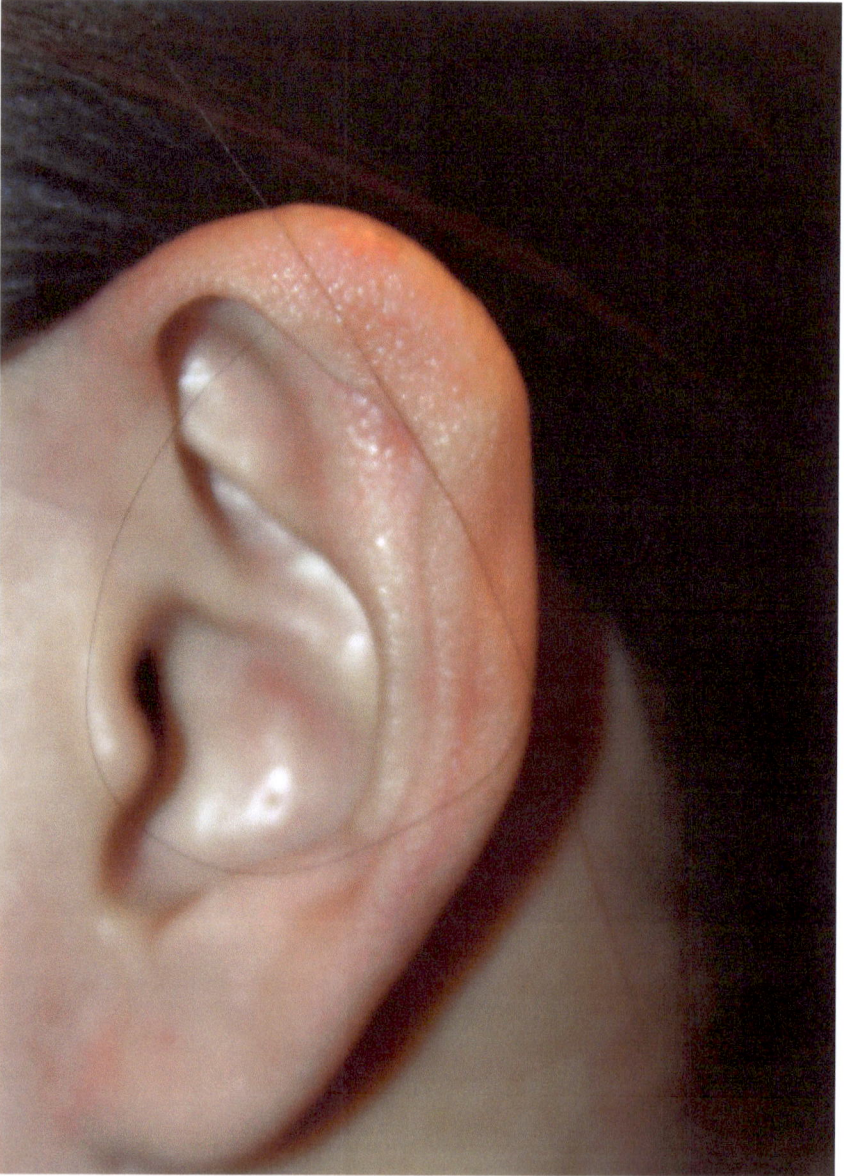

Fig. 119: Same patient as shown in *Fig 117*, follow up eighteen months later.

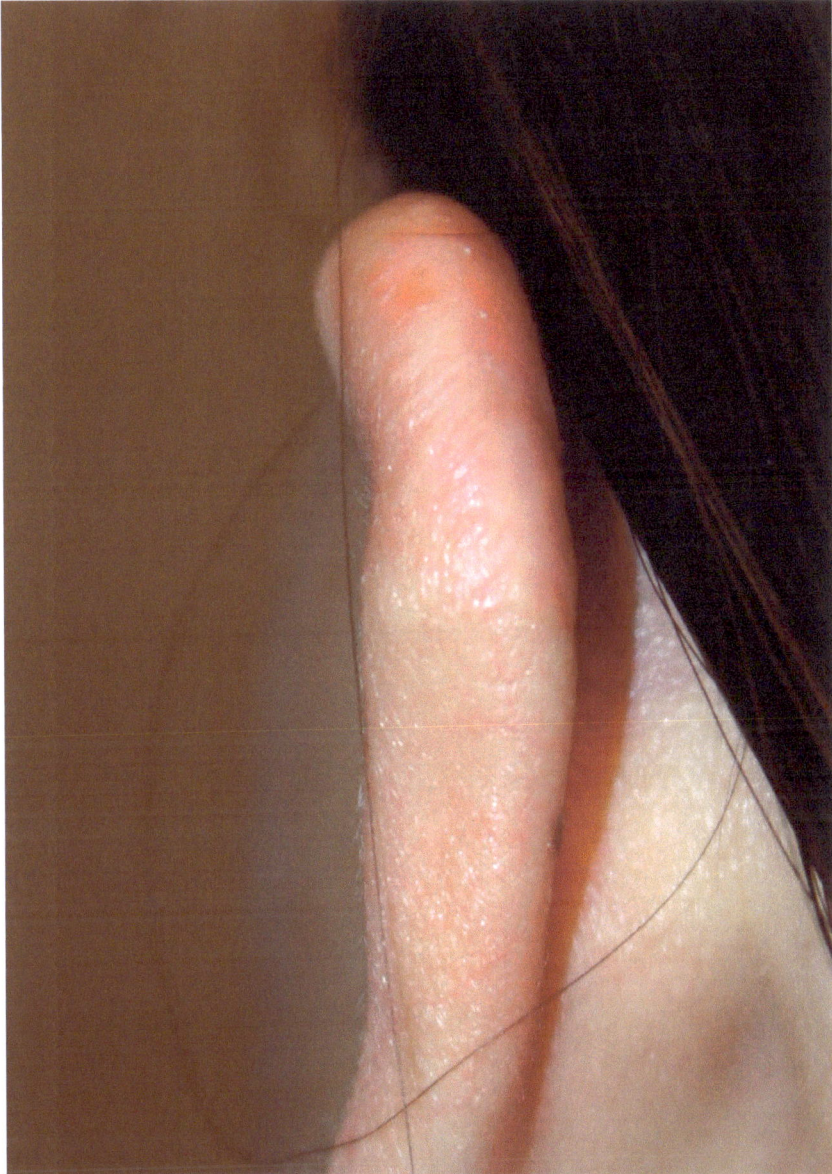

Fig. 120: Same patient as shown in *Fig 117*, follow up eighteen months later.

10 TREATMENT OF SECONDAY EAR KELOIDS

UNDER NO CIRCUMSTANCES should any patient undergo a second keloid surgery for the removal of a recurrent keloid. Surgery will almost always make secondary keloids worse and almost unanimously results in loss of ear tissue and disfigurement. Secondary ear keloids should only be treated with cryotherapy. Cryotherapy can effectively reduce the mass of secondary keloids. For those whose keloids are still not too large, cryotherapy often results in normalization of ear anatomy.

As compared to small secondary keloids, large secondary ear keloids tend to have a higher relapse rate after cryotherapy. As a general rule, the smaller the secondary keloid is, the better the outcome.

Massive secondary ear keloids tend to expand from the ear into the skin that surrounds the ear, either involving the face or the skin behind the ear. Treatment of these keloids is rather more challenging, will take a lot longer—often more than a year—and will require the intra-lesional injection of chemotherapy drugs, in addition to cryotherapy.

Much like secondary keloids, under no circumstances should otoplasty induced keloids be treated with yet another surgery. Surgery will almost always make otoplasty keloids worse and almost always results in the formation of a larger keloid. These keloids should primarily be treated with cryotherapy. Facelift-induced keloids often require multi-modality treatment, using cryotherapy and intra-lesional steroids or chemotherapy.

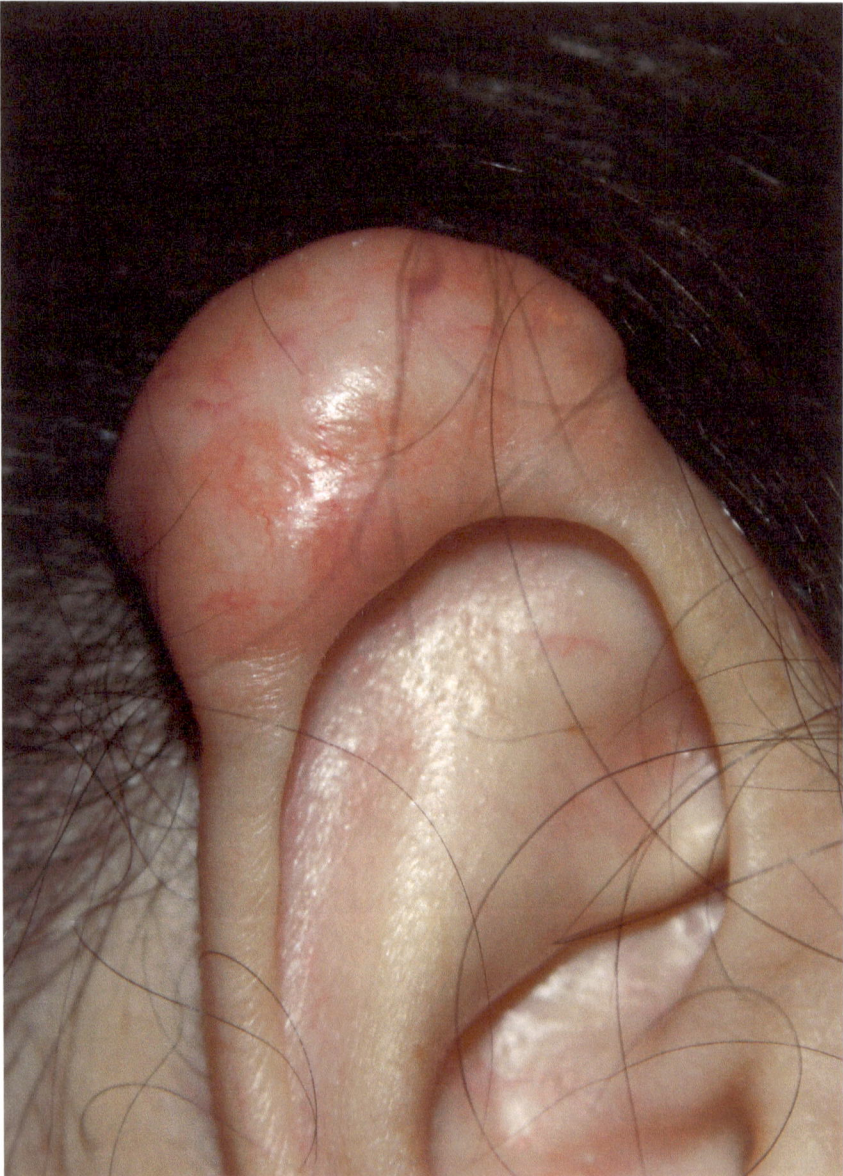

Fig. 121: Disfiguring recurrence of keloid in the helix of ear. This keloid has been resistant to prior surgeries, as well as steroids. Like many other women with similar issues, this patient always kept her hair down, or wore a hat in order to conceal the unsightly appearance of her keloid.

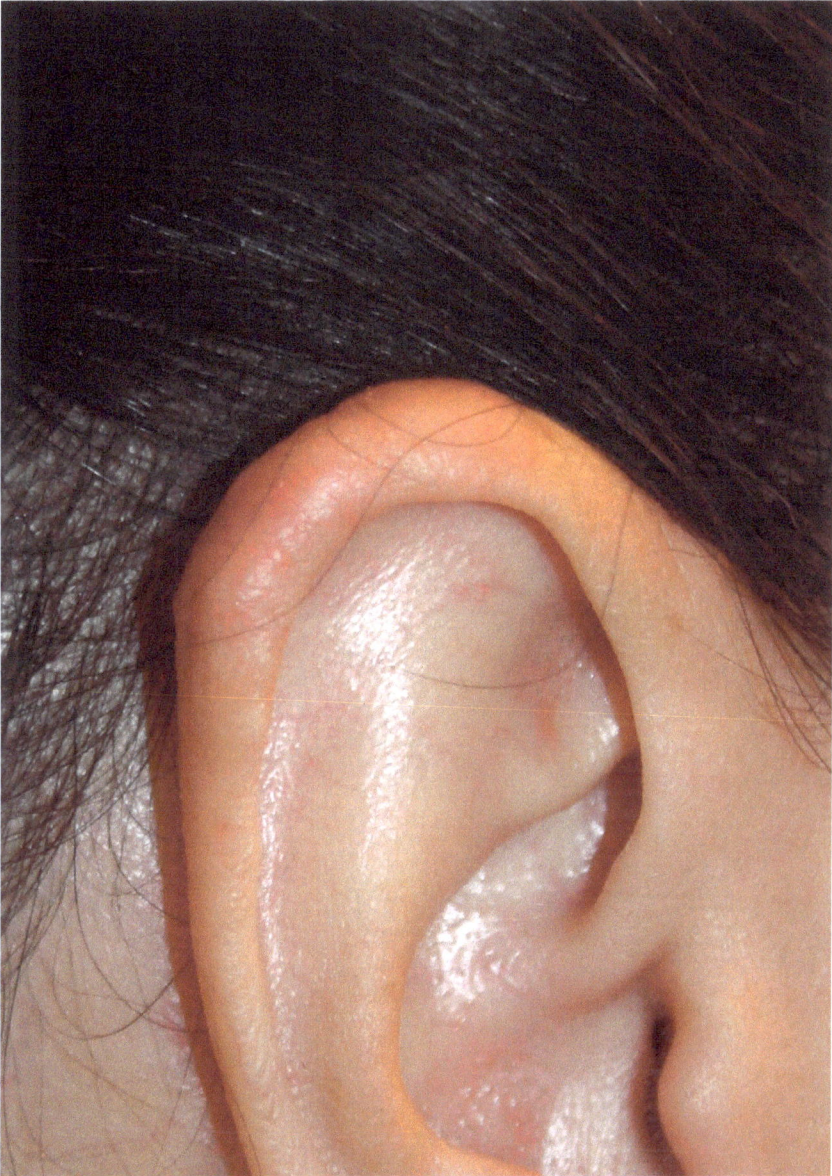

Fig. 122: Eighteen month follow up of the patient depicted in *Fig 121*. Treating this secondary keloid required several courses of cryotherapy and intra-lesional steroids/chemotherapy.

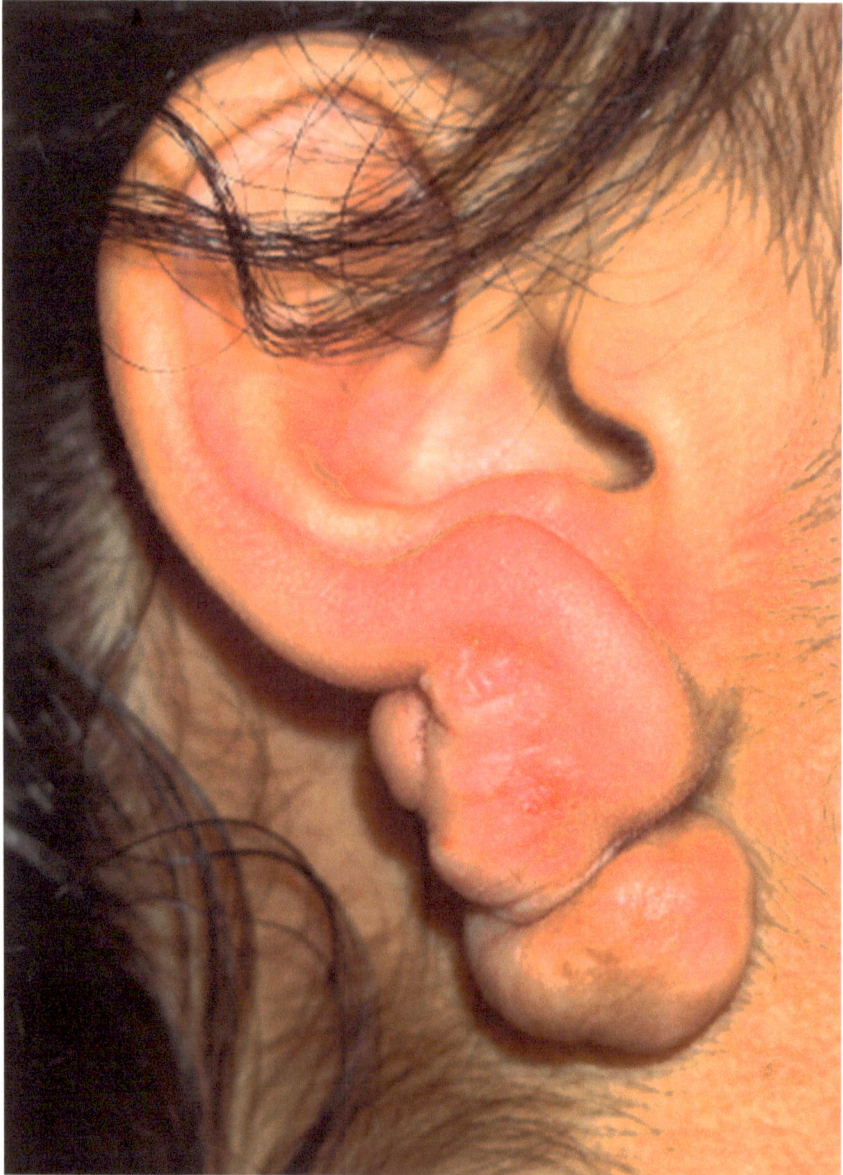

Fig. 123: Disfiguring recurrence of an earlobe keloid in a young woman. This keloid has been resistant to prior surgeries as well as steroids.

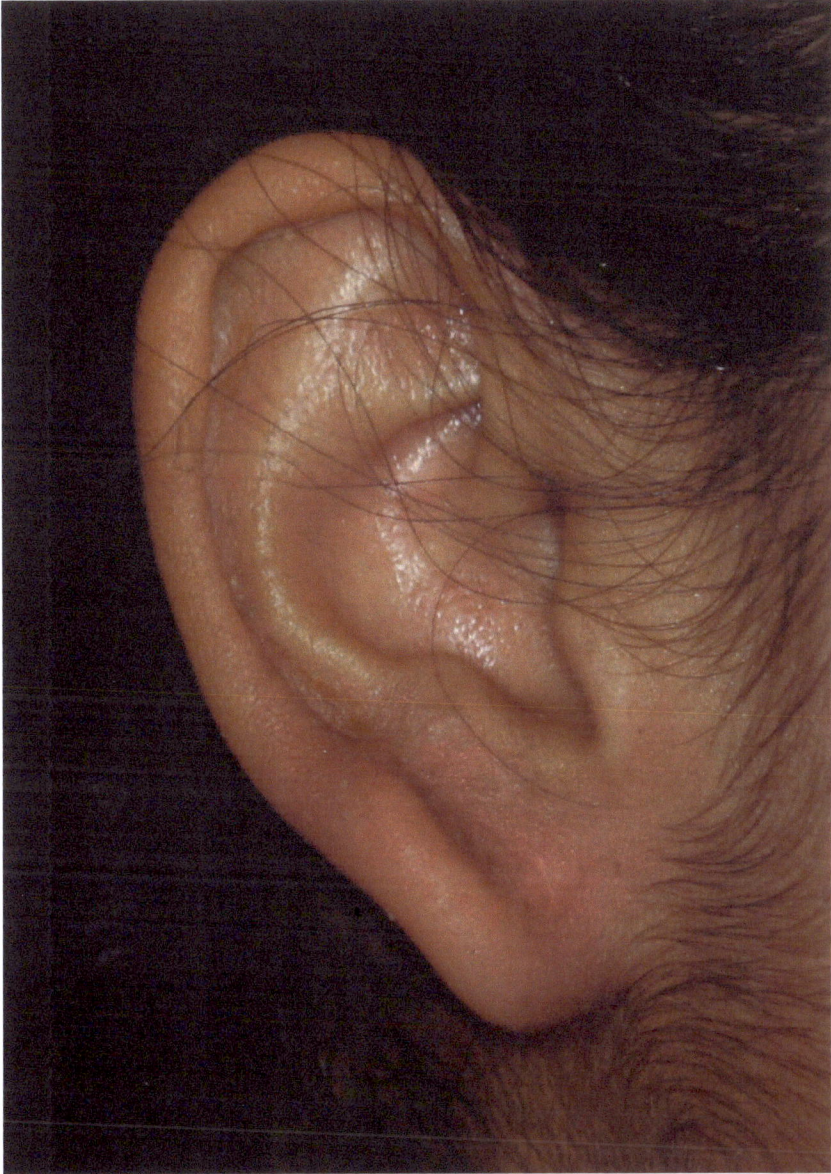

Fig. 124: Nine-month follow up of the patient depicted in *Fig 123*. This complex secondary keloid only required several courses of cryotherapy.

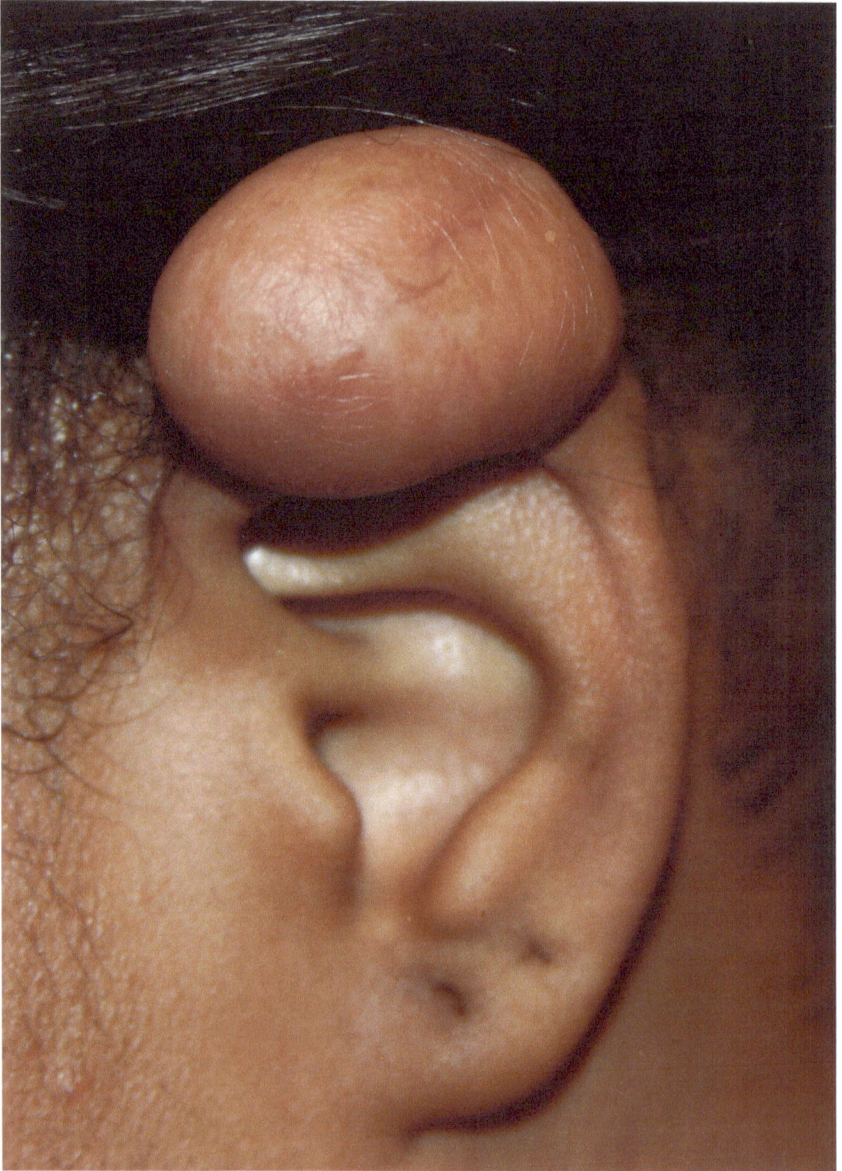

Fig. 125: Secondary ear keloid in a young woman.

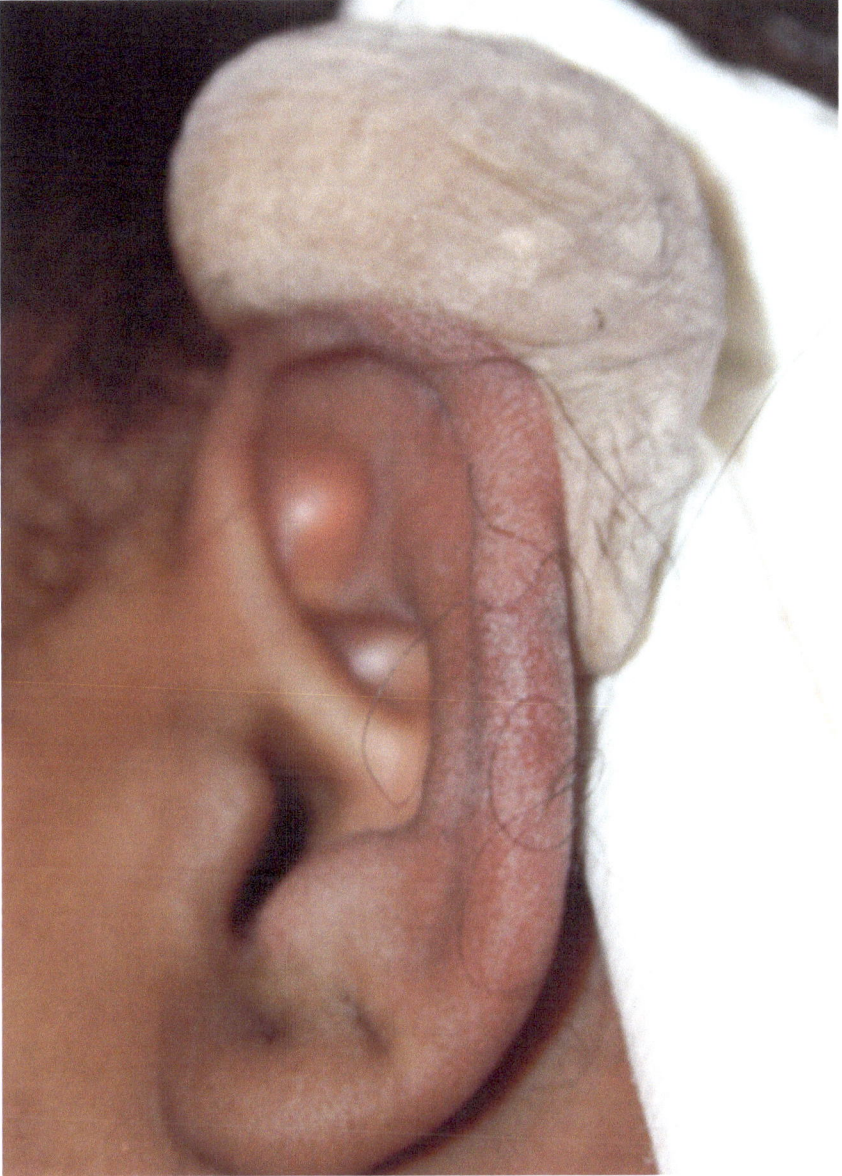

Fig. 126: Secondary ear keloid immediately after cryotherapy, same patient as shown in *Fig. 125*. The frozen keloid appears white.

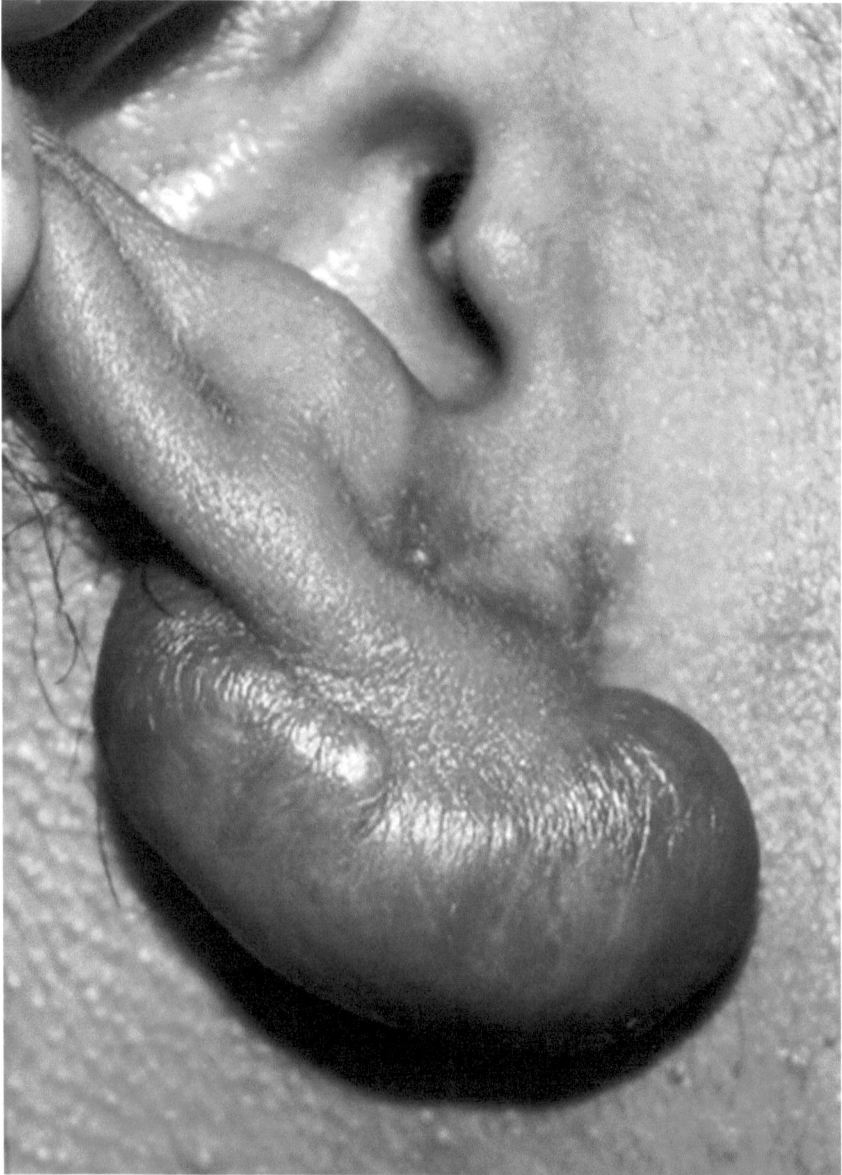

Fig. 127: Secondary earlobe keloid.

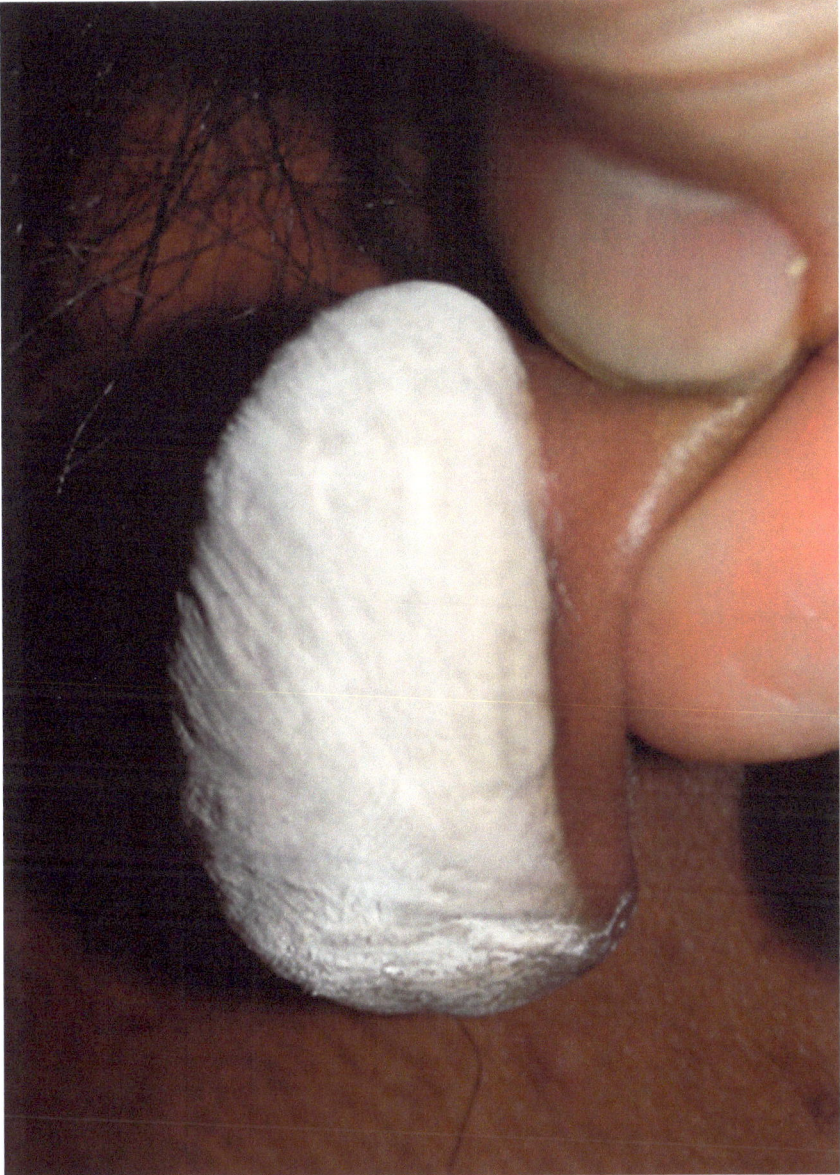

Fig. 128: Secondary earlobe immediately after cryotherapy, same patient shown in *Fig. 127.* The frozen keloid appears white.

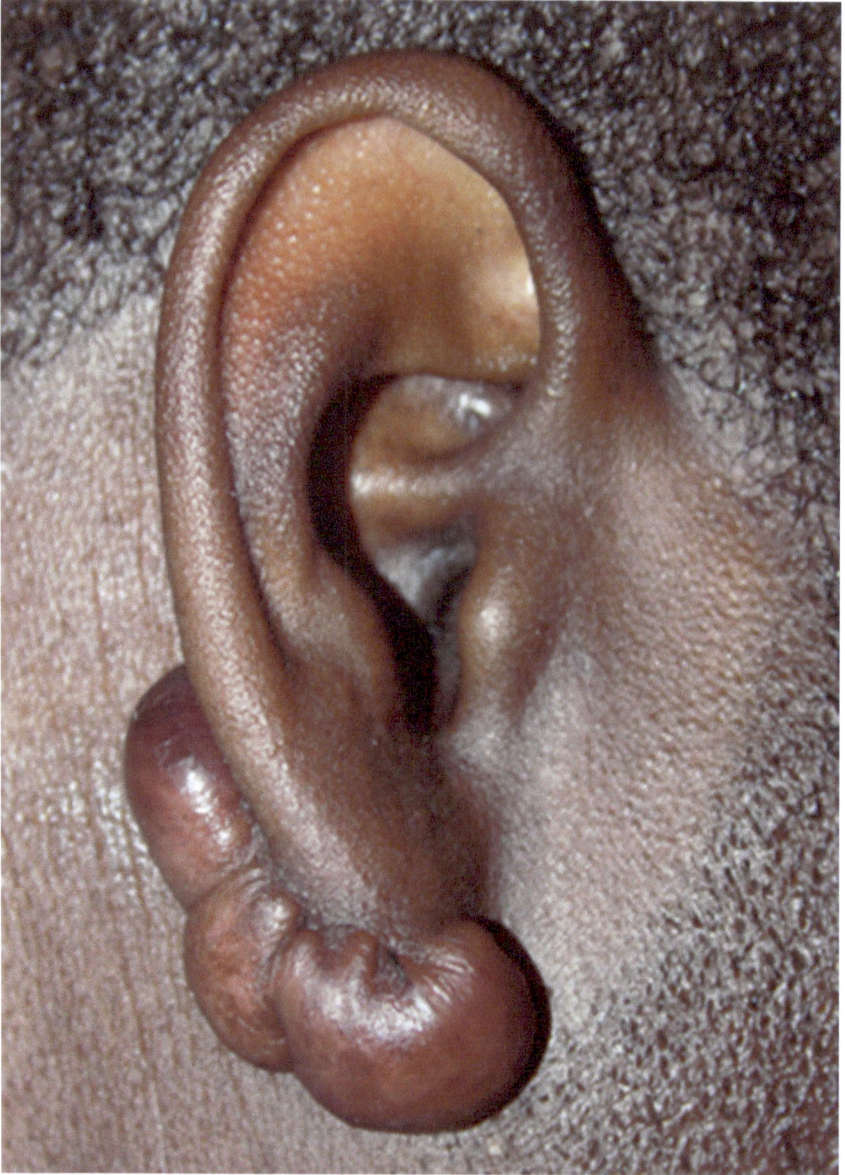

Fig. 129: Secondary ear keloid.

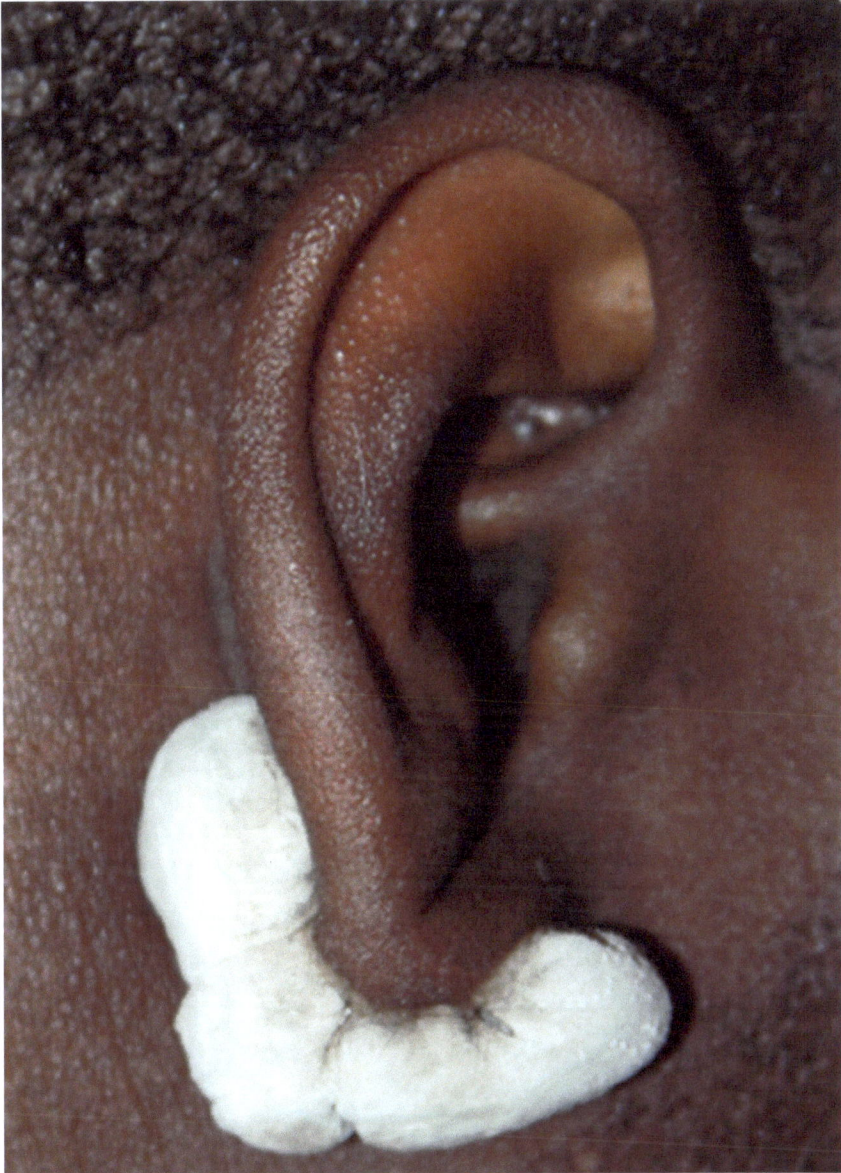

Fig. 130: Secondary earlobe keloid immediately after cryotherapy, same patient shown in *Fig. 129*. Note that topical cryotherapy can easily be conformed to the unique shape of the keloid. The frozen keloid appears white.

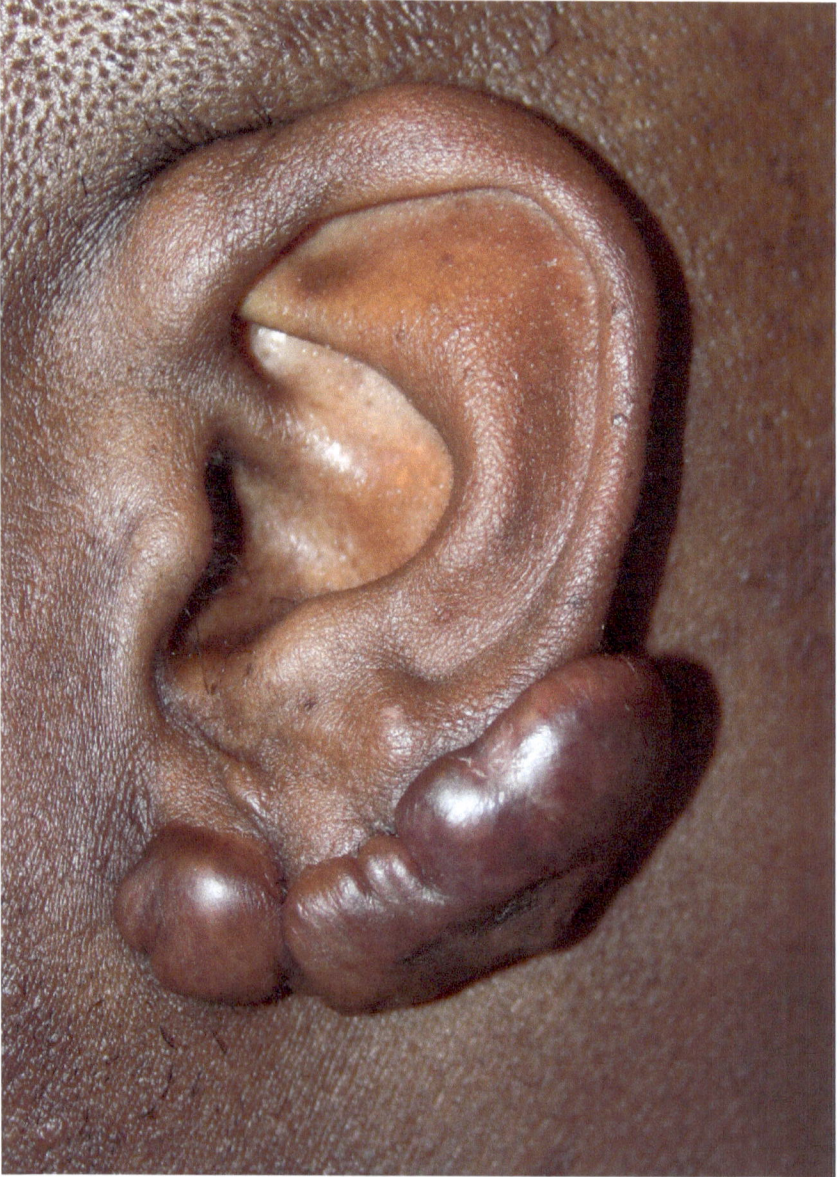

Fig. 131: Secondary earlobe keloid.

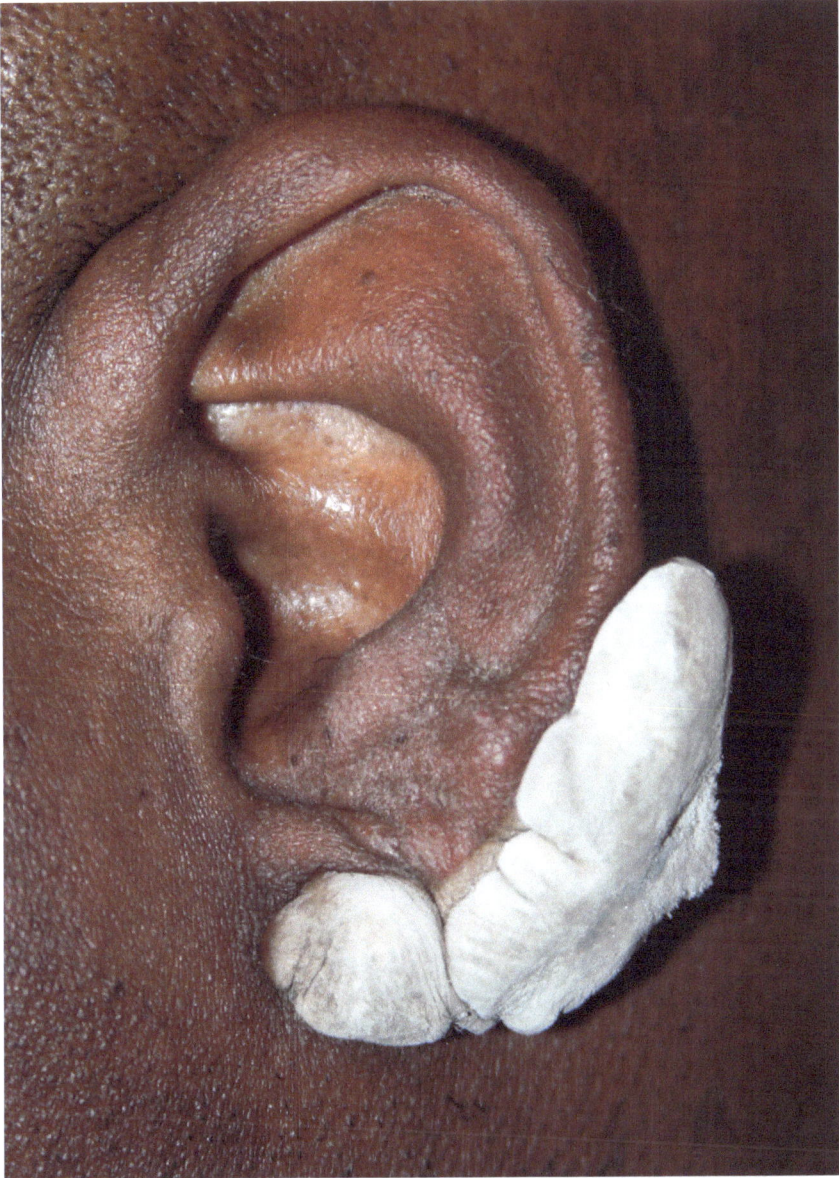

Fig. 132: Secondary earlobe keloid immediately after cryotherapy, same patient shown in *Fig. 131*. The frozen keloid appears white.

11 HARMFUL TREATMENTS

EAR BANDING IS a home remedy that some patients choose to apply on their own for the treatment of ear keloids.

The therapeutic principal behind this method is that the tight elastic band, or other material that might be used, would reduce blood flow to the keloid and result in tissue necrosis.

Although the method can work and induce keloid necrosis, the process may induce necrosis of normal ear tissue beyond the boundaries of the keloid itself, or may not induce enough pressure, and therefore be totally ineffective.

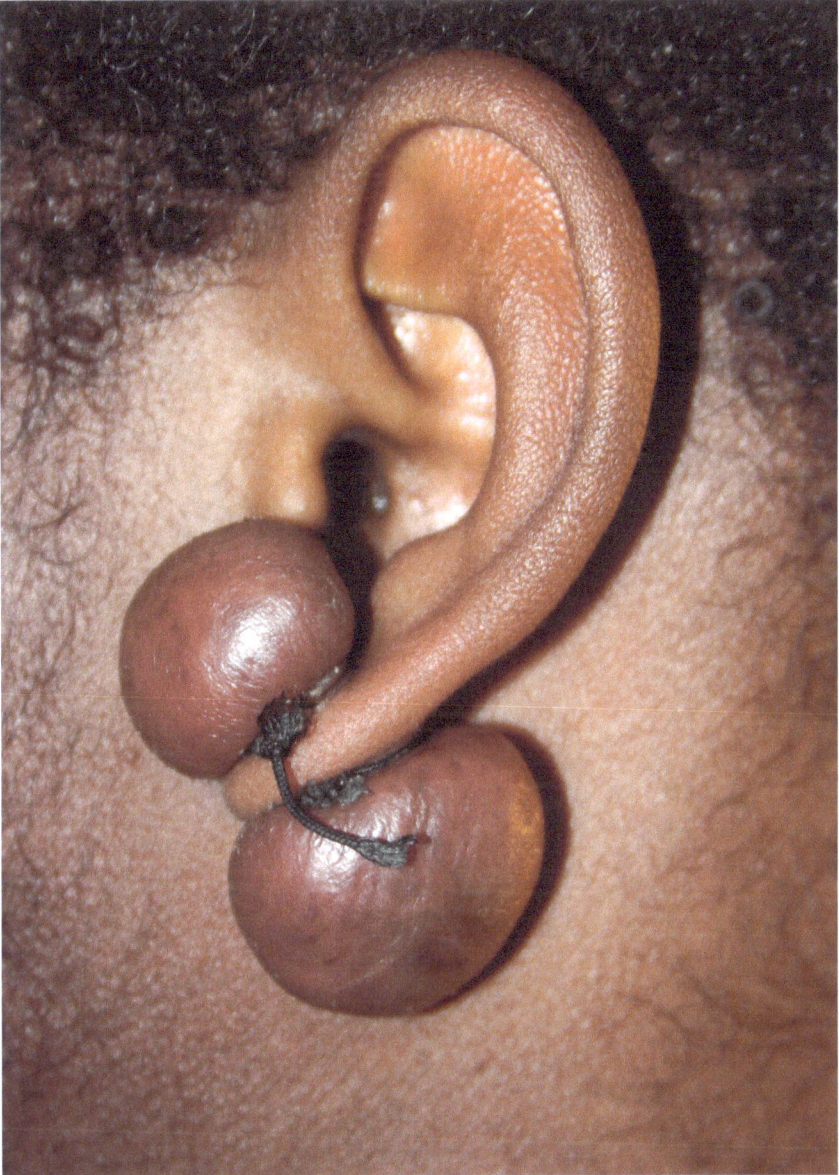

Fig. 133. Ear bands applied to two earlobe keloids without any effect.

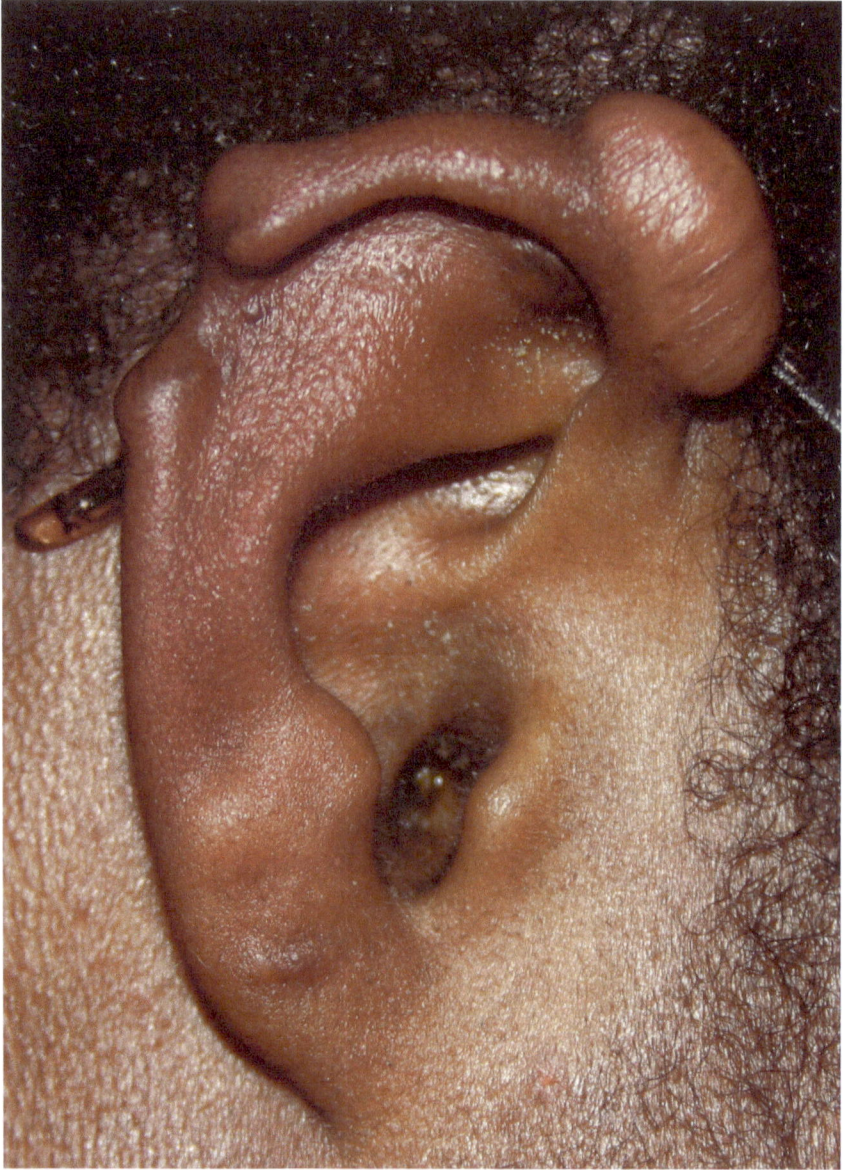

Fig. 134 Loss of normal ear helix from ear banding.

About the Author

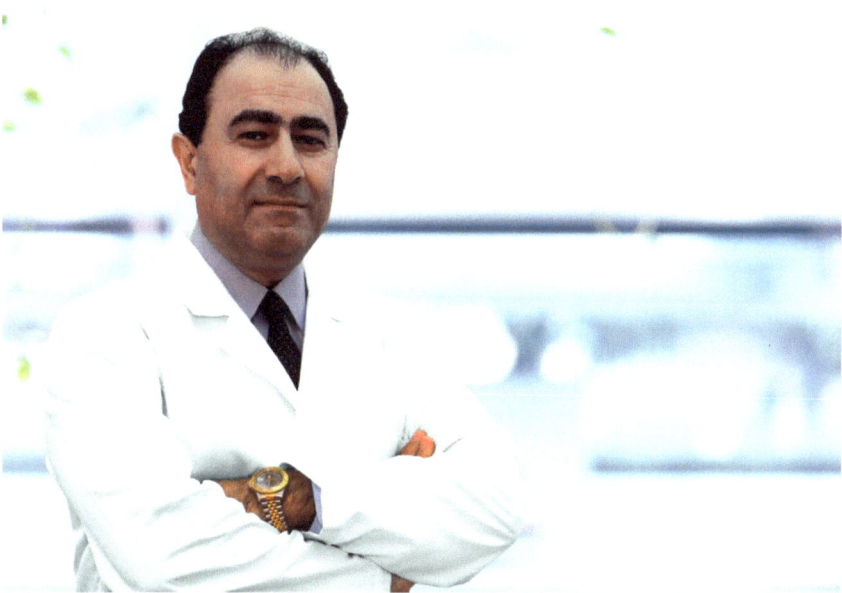

MICHAEL H. TIRGAN, MD is a medical oncologist who specializes in the treatment and research of keloid disorder. He began seeing keloid patients through his oncology practice and soon realized the need for highly trained specialists to treat this deeply misunderstood and complex disorder of the skin.

In 2008, Dr. Tirgan began focusing his practice on the non-surgical treatment of keloid and now is the only physician in North America with a pure specialty practice that is limited solely to the treatment of individuals with this disorder. He has treated approximately 900 keloid patients, adults and children, with all types of keloid.

He is an avid researcher of keloid and has published peer-reviewed articles on his findings. His dedication and sole focus on helping keloid patients, coupled with his vast clinical experience, have allowed him to develop unparalleled expertise in treating this complicated disorder.

Dr. Tirgan is an attending physician at Mount Sinai St. Luke's Roosevelt Hospital and Rockefeller University Hospital in New York, NY. He is also a clinical instructor at the Icahn School of Medicine at Mount Sinai.

www.ingramcontent.com/pod-product-compliance
Lightning Source LLC
Chambersburg PA
CBHW041306210326
41598CB00011B/857